Control of

Gastrointestinal

Function

MODERN CONCEPTS IN MEDICAL PHYSIOLOGY

A MACMILLAN SERIES

Lysle H. Peterson, M.D., Consulting Editor

Frank P. Brooks, M.D., Sc.D. (Med.)

ASSOCIATE PROFESSOR OF MEDICINE AND OF PHYSIOLOGY
UNIVERSITY OF PENNSYLVANIA SCHOOL OF MEDICINE
CHIEF, GASTROINTESTINAL CLINIC
HOSPITAL OF THE UNIVERSITY OF PENNSYLVANIA

Control of Gastrointestinal Function

AN INTRODUCTION TO THE PHYSIOLOGY OF THE GASTROINTESTINAL TRACT

The Macmillan Company | Collier-Macmillan Limited, London

18/2/70

First Printing, 1970

Library of Congress catalog card number: 70–80786

THE MACMILLAN COMPANY
866 THIRD AVENUE, NEW YORK, NEW YORK 10022
COLLIER-MACMILLAN CANADA, LTD., TORONTO, ONTARIO

Printed in the United States of America

To Emily, Bill, Sally, and Robert

in appreciation of their patience and encouragement

Preface

THIS BRIEF TEXTBOOK HIGHLIGHTS those aspects of gastrointestinal physiology that are of greatest significance in clinical medicine. The organization is based on the major functions of the gastrointestinal tract—that is, secretion, digestion, absorption, and motility. Within each major function, the contributions of specific portions of the digestive tract are considered in the usual aboral sequence.

In general, cellular processes are considered first. A particular attempt has been made to relate structure, as determined by electron and light microscopy, to function. Also included are discussions of the periods of growth and development of the gut, which contribute to one's understanding of function and which have particular significance in pediatric practice; the adaptive changes, which are presently of considerable clinical interest; the role of cellular transport in various secretory and absorptive processes; the differentiation of water and electrolytes, and macromolecules such as proteins, polypeptides, and mucopolysaccharides; bioelectric phenomena, which are involved in most digestive functions; and some of the techniques available for examination of function.

Following the material on cellular mechanisms is a description of what each component of the gastrointestinal system does and the rate at which a particular process occurs. This leads logically into a discussion of control of the system by endocrine glands and autonomic nervous system, and, most importantly, by release of homoral agents during nervous stimulation. When appropriate, studies in man and clinical correlations are emphasized, and the subject is examined from the viewpoint of systems analysis. Examples of pathophysiology and pertinent illustrations are included throughout, and a summary of significant physiologic knowledge is located at the end of each chapter. References, which also appear after each chapter, serve a twofold purpose: to document various statements within the body of the text, and to lead the reader with sufficient time and motivation to more detailed discussions of various aspects of gastrointestinal physiology.

Control of Gastrointestinal Function is designed as a concise summary of physiologic principles for students in various phases of the present-day medical curriculum, from the first-year "core" course to the clinical clerkships in internal medicine, surgery, and gastroenterology; for graduate students in various biomedical disciplines; for house officers and postdoctoral fellows; and for practicing physicians in the fields of internal medicine, pediatrics, gastroenterology, abdominal surgery, and general surgery.

The author wishes to acknowledge the assistance of Drs. John R. Brobeck, Irwin M. Arias, Robert Crane, and Charles Tidball, who reviewed portions of the final version of the manuscript and offered valuable comments and criticisms; Dr. George Karreman, who helped plan the model of enterohepatic circulation; and Dr. Lysle H. Peterson, consulting editor of the *Modern Concepts in Medical Physiology* series, who provided this opportunity to participate in a stimulating educational venture.

Frank P. Brooks

Contents

Control of Gastrointestinal Function

Introduction

THE MAJOR FUNCTIONS of the gastrointestinal tract are the digestion of food, accomplished in part by the secretions of the digestive glands; the absorption from the intestinal lumen; and the movement of intestinal contents through the alimentary tract. Each portion of the organ system appears to contain the mechanisms necessary to accomplish its function within itself, free of extrinsic nervous or humoral control. This is illustrated dramatically by the ability of the isolated in vitro stomach to secrete, the everted gut sac to absorb, and the isolated intestinal segment to contract. In some instances function can be localized more specifically, as to the smooth muscle of the guinea pig taenia coli, free of ganglion cells, or to the small intestinal mucosa, free of the muscularis propria. As yet collections of single cell types have been difficult to obtain for physiologic studies, but homogenates and fragments of tissue are in common use. Slowly, knowledge accumulates on how these cells or organs control their activity. The control of function in the intact mammal involves many more variables, including the whole area of the behavioral sciences. Nonetheless, behaviorists and systems-analysis-minded biologists and neurophysiologists are finding this a challenging field. For the physician dealing with the prevention, diagnosis, and treatment of gastrointestinal illness, it would appear to be a major need for establishing a rational basis of action.

Probably the control of food intake represents a prime example of how these various fields of study can be brought to bear upon problems of control and regulation. The role of the gastrointestinal tract in this system has usually been minimized. The failure of gastrectomy or vagotomy to modify certain experimental models for the control of food intake and similarly to disturb the maintenance of a steady body weight in man has been taken to indicate that the alimentary tract is of little importance. However, the failure to influence a function by removal of an organ may reflect primarily the compensatory mechanisms of the remaining system rather than a lack of function of the removed part.

We know that single afferent fibers in the vagus nerve exhibit action potentials in response to mechanical stimulation of the stomach and coincident with contractions of the gastric wall (11).° Therefore the central nervous system receives information on the state of the gastric musculature. In man, the hunger pang, which can be correlated with large-amplitude contractions of the stomach, disappears after vagotomy (14). In animals with gastric fistulas, the inhibition of oral food intake is related to the volume of a meal introduced directly into the stomach. When meals of over 20 per cent of the volume of control meals were introduced 20 minutes before mealtime, compensatory decreases in oral food intake occurred, even when inert material was substituted for food. This suggests that gastric distention may act as a major signal for the cessation of feeding.

Rats are able to regulate food intake when fed directly into the stomach (4). However, when choices of food to be eaten must be made, when incentives are necessary to stimulate food intake, and when feeding behavior must be aroused and sustained, then oropharyngeal factors become important. Taste and smell play the most important roles under these circumstances. They are also the basis for many dietary habits in man.

Water intake has a somewhat similar control system. Dryness of the mouth is considered as a factor influencing water intake. Removal of the salivary glands or ligating the ducts in rats results in increased water intake. On a dry diet this may amount to a doubling of the amount of water. Furthermore the pattern of drinking changes; the rats drink in short periods of licking immediately after taking the dry food into their mouth.

Therefore, it is reasonable to conclude that the upper gastrointestinal tract under normal circumstances does play a part in the control of food and water intake.

From the point of view of total body function, the gastrointestinal tract has an important influence on several other body functions. The gut serves as a reservoir for blood and extracellular fluid. Strictly speaking, the fluid in the lumen of the intestine is outside the body, but it can readily exchange both water and solute. Table 1-1 shows the exchangeable sodium, potassium, and chloride in lumen of the gastrointestinal tract of rabbits expressed in absolute amounts and as a percentage of the total. The greater percentage of exchangeable ions and body water was in the cecum and transverse colon (3,8,20).

The relationships between the circulatory system and the gastrointestinal

_____

°Parenthetical numbers pertain to References at the end of the chapter.

TABLE 1-1
Distribution of Water and Electrolytes in the Lumen of the Gastrointestinal Tract of Rabbits

	Stomach	Small Intestine	Cecum and Transverse Colon	"Total" GI Tract
		Amount (mEq)		
Sodium	0.8 ± 0.4	3.1 ± 1.1	10.0 ± 2.0	13.7 ± 2.4
Potassium	0.7 ± 0.3	1.2 ± 0.4	4.5 ± 3.1	7.1 ± 2.8
Chloride	8.7 ± 3.4	1.8 ± 0.4	1.2 ± 0.3	11.8 ± 3.6
		Per Cent of Exchangeable Ion		
Sodium	0.9 ± 0.4	3.2 ± 1.2	10.2 ± 2.1	14.2 ± 2.4
Potassium	0.7 ± 0.3	1.2 ± 0.4	4.5 ± 2.7	7.2 ± 2.2
Chloride	11.7 ± 4.4	2.5 ± 0.7	1.7 ± 0.4	16.0 ± 4.5
		Amount (ml)		
Water	65 ± 15	31 ± 12	93 ± 22	189 ± 40
		Per Cent of Total Body Water		
Water	4.1 ± 0.9	2.0 ± 1.0	6.0 ± 1.6	12.1 ± 2.7

tract are difficult to define. Eating initiates an increase in blood flow to the gut, but this occurs as a part of an increase in cardiac output and the percentage reaching the intestine does not change (9). After implanting electromagnetic flowmeters on the superior mesenteric artery in dogs, significant increases in blood flow one hour after eating were found which could not be accounted for by an increased cardiac output (24).

Measurements of total blood flow to the gut may be misleading, since in many cases only one component of the organ may be affected and a compensatory change in the other tissues may leave the total blood flow unchanged. Techniques for determining mucosal blood flow in a quantitative fashion have been difficult to devise, especially those that could be applied to conscious animals (12).

The intestine is said to exhibit an autoregulation of blood flow. This means that flow remains constant in the face of changes in blood pressure, since the rise or fall of the latter is countered by an appropriate change in vascular resistance (17).

The gastrointestinal tract is an important factor in protein synthesis and catabolism. The pancreas and small intestinal mucosa are among the sites of most rapid protein synthesis in the body, and the intestine is considered by some to be the major site of the degradation of plasma protein albumin. Small amounts of albumin have been found in the secretions of the digestive glands under normal circumstances. The rapid shedding of cells lining the intestine contributes up to 50 gm of protein per day in man (19).

The metabolic functions of the liver are predicated upon an ample supply of nutriment via the portal vein, while the postprandial accumulation of chylomicrons in blood is the result of the entrance of lymph from the small intestine. Studies of the comparatively greater release of insulin following oral glucose compared to intravenous glucose implicate a gastrointestinal hormone (26).

The control of cholesterol synthesis resides in part in the intestine. While hepatic cholesterologenesis varies with the intake of cholesterol, the small intestinal rate of cholesterol synthesis varies inversely with amount of bile salts in the intestinal lumen. Diversion of bile or binding of bile salts with cholestyramine results in a marked increase in intestinal cholesterologenesis without change in the synthesis of cholesterol by the liver (1).

Pathophysiology

Depletion of intestinal content or glandular secretions can have profound systemic effects. Pyloric stenosis with attendant vomiting results in alkalosis and hypokalemia, which under extreme conditions may lead to the development of tetany and cardiac arrhythmias. Cholera may result in truly massive depletion (27). Figure 1-1 shows a successfully treated patient surrounded by the bottles of intravenous fluids needed to restore his fluid balance. This occurs in the face of normal intestinal epithelium. Presumably there is a malfunction of the submucosal capillaries. An equally devastating diarrhea may occur with a pancreatic islet-cell adenoma (7). Here the mechanism is thought to be mediated by a polypeptide produced by the tumor.

Excessive loss of albumin into the gut in patients with constrictive pericarditis and an increased venous pressure may produce severe hypoproteinemia with the anticipated consequences of edema and ascites. This phenomenon, which can be quantitated with radioactive tracers, has the rather formidable designation of protein-losing gastroenteropathy (16).

Radiation exposure in large amounts is associated with diarrhea and sometimes septicemia with the gut as a portal of entry because the high rate of cellular turnover makes the intestinal epithelium particularly sensitive (29). Similarly, intestinal obstruction with loss of the barrier function of the intestinal mucosa permits bacteria to enter the splanchnic venous drainage.

Endocrinopathies may have predominantly gastrointestinal manifestations. Hypopituitarism leads to atrophic changes in the digestive tract, but anorexia nervosa and starvation may lead to secondary hypopituitarism (18). Adrenocortical insufficiency may present with diarrhea, anorexia, and weight loss. The epithelium of the gut participates in the inability to retain sodium and also exhibits mild malabsorption of fat (23).

The development of impaired liver function interferes with the normal removal or modification of constituents of the portal blood. Ammonia produced by intestinal bacteria gains access to the peripheral circulation and probably

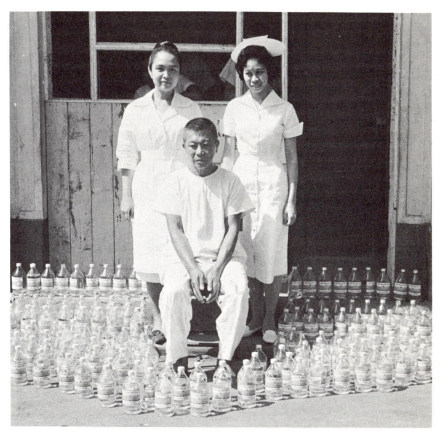

FIGURE 1-1.   A 53-kilogram patient convalescing from cholera, shown with enough bottles to provide the nearly 80 liters of intravenous electrolyte solutions that were required to maintain his body fluids during five days of diarrhea due to cholera. (Official U.S. Navy photograph, obtained through the courtesy of Dr. R. A. Phillips, and R. H. Watten of U.S. Naval Medical Research Unit No. 2.)

plays an important role in the development of hepatic coma (6). Dietary protein when absorbed as amino acids under these circumstances escapes the liver and leads to the "meat intoxication" first seen in dogs with portacaval shunts in Pavlov's laboratory.

These examples should serve to emphasize the close relationship between the gastrointestinal tract and the function of other organ systems in health and disease.

The particular emphasis of this book lies in the control of digestive function. Control may be exerted at the cellular level, upon a specific tissue such as the intestinal epithelium, upon an entire organ or even the entire gastrointestinal tract. Cellular control is presently being studied as a genetic problem, through protein synthesis or as an effect on cell membranes (2,15). Figure

1-2 illustrates current conceptions of the control of protein synthesis. Note that three types of ribonucleic acid are involved—messenger RNA, transfer RNA, and ribosomal RNA. Genetic repression with gene activation and reproduction of genetic information leads to increased production of RNA and the production of specific proteins. Characteristic of this kind of cellular control is its inhibition by actinomycin D and puromycin. The former interferes with RNA synthesis, and the latter with protein synthesis (10).

Hormonal or neurohumoral control of cellular function is thought in a number of instances to act through a direct effect on cell membranes. The enzyme adenyl cyclase, upon activation by hormones, is thought to form 3,5-adenosine monophosphate (AMP) from adenopyrophosphate. A variety of

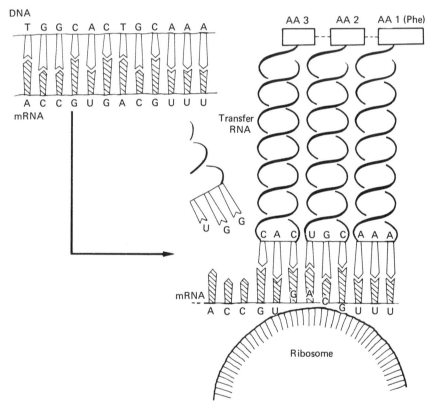

FIGURE 1-2. Current scheme of the mechanism of protein synthesis. Complementary messenger RNA (mRNA) is first formed on DNA. Following this it attaches to the ribosomes. Then the base groups of the mRNA are paired with the complementary base groups of transfer RNA's which are carrying activated amino acids. Finally, the amino acids are joined together to form the polypeptide chain. (From P. Karlson. *Introduction to Modern Biochemistry.* New York: Academic Press, 1965.)

secretory cells have been found to secrete coincident with an increased amount of cyclic AMP formation (28).

At the organ level, control of function resides with the local autonomic nervous system and possibly with so-called local hormones of unknown significance such as serotonin, kinins, substance P, and darmstoff. In general, cellular functions *may* occur independently of such mechanisms, as in the case of "spontaneous" secretion of certain salivary glands, transport by intestinal epithelium, and contractions of intestinal smooth muscle. However, activities requiring coordinated functions, such as the peristaltic reflex, are dependent upon local reflex pathways of the autonomic nervous system.

Finally, in the normal intact organism the gut is subject to the full complexity of control exerted through the central nervous system and endocrine glands. In order to apply the full rigor of current systems analysis it is necessary to determine the variable that is regulated, to alter the variable and observe the response, and to identify the components involved with their own particular characteristics. From here one can proceed to testing a model. According to one group of distinguished physiologists, this almost always involves the use of a computer (22). An attempt has been made to apply a mathematical approach to the control of the enterohepatic circulation of bile salts. This is presented in the final chapter of the book.

As in the case of other biologic systems, the gastrointestinal system is complicated in the sense that it has many inputs and outputs. There are also complex interactions between the several subsystems and their processes and mechanisms. Figure 1-3 illustrates these relationships.

A promising approach for better understanding of any of the subsystems as parts of the whole system is, as mentioned, that of systems analysis, using computers. This may lead to more quantitative relationships, which are required for further progress in the field, and is in keeping with current trends in physiology and pathophysiology. Such developments may result in a better understanding of processes in health and disease.

In addition to quantitative data, the search for such relationships will uncover many gaps in our present knowledge and suggest the design of new experiments. Such are the reasons for the systems approach, which seems destined to play an increasingly important role in the future of gastrointestinal physiology.

Many practical problems remain in the application of a systems analysis approach. In gastrointestinal physiology it has been difficult to identify the regulated variables. There are a few candidates—the hydrogen ion concentration of the pyloric antrum and the small intestine, the tension of intestinal smooth muscle, and the tonicity of intestinal content. However, in an organ system that, in our society, is called upon to function at a maximal level three times a day at mealtime and to subside into inactivity during eight hours of sleep, it is not surprising that controlling factors in the environment acting through nerves and hormones seem to overpower the local system. I am aware

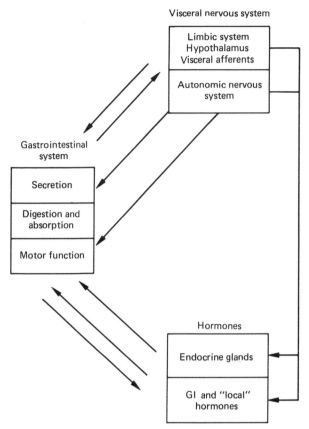

FIGURE 1-3.

of only a few experiments in digestive physiology that follow the foregoing demands. These include the study of the catabolism of plasma proteins by compartmental analysis (5), the behavior of the blood pepsinogen (25), and the relationship between contraction and electrical activity in the small bowel (21). For the most part, we shall have to construct signal flow pathways and components into an operational diagram showing the connectivity of the system. Perhaps this will be sufficient for those who must treat the perturbations of the system in disease. Until now it has been difficult to see how systems analysis has modified patient care in those organ systems where it has been most successfully applied. Doubtless similar objections have been offered to every attempt to apply physicochemical laws to medicine.

References

1. Dietschy, J. M. The role of bile salts in controlling the rate of intestinal cholesterologenesis. *J. Clin. Invest.* **47**: 286–300, 1968.

2. Edelman, I. S., R. Bogoroch, and G. A. Porter. On the mechanism of action of aldosterone on sodium transport: The role of protein synthesis. *Proc. Nat. Acad. Sci. USA* **50:** 1169–1176, 1963.

3. Edelman, I. S., and N. J. Sweet. Gastrointestinal water and electrolytes. I. The equilibration of radiosodium in gastrointestinal contents and the proportion of exchangeable sodium (Na_e) in the gastrointestinal tract. *J. Clin. Invest.* **35:** 502–511, 1956.

4. Epstein, A. N. Oropharyngeal factors in feeding and drinking. In: *Handbook of Physiology*. Section 6: Alimentary Tract. Vol. I: Control of Food and Water Intake. Edited by C. F. Code. Washington, D.C.: American Physiological Society, 1967, pp. 197–218.

5. Franks, J. J. Calculation of the albumin catabolic rate in the non-steady state. *J. Gen. Physiol.* **46:** 405–413, 1962–63.

6. Gabuzda, G. J. Ammonia metabolism and hepatic coma. *Gastroenterology* **53:** 806–810, 1967.

7. Gardner, J. D., and J. J. Cerda. In vitro inhibition of intestinal fluid and electrolyte transfer by a non-beta islet cell tumor. *Proc. Soc. Exp. Biol. Med.* **123:** 361–364, 1966.

8. Gotch, F., J. Nadell, and I. S. Edelman. Gastrointestinal water and electrolytes. IV. The equilibration of deuterium oxide (D_2O) in gastrointestinal contents and the proportion of total body water (TBW) in the gastrointestinal tract. *J. Clin. Invest.* **36:** 289–296, 1957.

9. Grim, E. The flow of blood in the mesenteric vessels. In: *Handbook of Physiology*. Section 2: Circulation. Vol. II. Edited by W. F. Hamilton. Washington, D.C.: American Physiological Society, 1963, pp. 1439–1456.

10. Hoaglund, M. B. Coding, information transfer, and protein synthesis. In: *The Metabolic Basis of Inherited Disease* (2nd. ed.). Edited by J. B. Stanbury, J. B. Wyngaarden, and D. S. Fredrickson. New York: McGraw-Hill Book Co., 1966, pp. 21–45.

11. Iggo, A. Gastroduodenal tension receptors with unmyelinated afferent fibers in the vagus of the cat. *Quart. J. Exp. Physiol.* **42:** 130–143, 1957.

12. Jacobson, E. D. Recent advances in the gastrointestinal circulation and related areas: comments on a symposium. *Gastroenterology* **52:** 332–337, 1967.

13. Jacobson, E. D., and T. J. Magnani. Some effects of hypophysectomy on gastrointestinal function and structure. *Gut* **5:** 473–479, 1964.

14. Janowitz, H. D. Role of the gastrointestinal tract in regulation of food intake. In: *Handbook of Physiology*. Section 6: Alimentary Tract. Vol. I: Food and Water Intake. Edited by C. F. Code. Washington, D.C.: American Physiology Society, 1967, pp. 219–224.

15. Janqueira, L. C. U. Control of cell secretion. In: *Secretory Mechanisms of Salivary Glands*. Edited by L. H. and C. A. Schneyer. New York: Academic Press, 1967, pp. 286–302.

16. Jarnum, S. *Protein-Losing Gastroenteropathy*. Philadelphia: F. A. Davis Co., 1963, pp. 26–30.

17. Johnson, P. O. Autoregulation of blood flow in the intestine. *Gastroenterology* **52:** 435–441, 1967.

18. McBrien, D. J., R. V. Jones, and B. Creamer. Steatorrhea in Addison's disease. *Lancet* **1:** 25–26, 1963.

19. Munro, H. N. Protein secretion into the gastrointestinal tract. In: *Postgraduate*

Gastro-Enterology. Edited by T. J. Thomson and I. E. Gillespie. London: Bailliere, Tindall and Cassell, 1966, pp. 58–67.

20. Nadell, J., N. J. Sweet, and I. S. Edelman. Gastrointestinal water and electrolytes. II. The equilibration of radiopotassium in gastrointestinal contents and the proportion of exchangeable potassium (K_e) in the gastrointestinal tract. *J. Clin. Invest.* **35:** 512–521, 1956.

21. Nelsen, T. S., and J. C. Becker. Simulation of the electrical and mechanical gradient of the small intestine. *Am. J. Physiol.* **214:** 749–757, 1968.

22. Physiology Training Committee. A view of systems physiology. *Physiologist* **11:** 115–133, 1968.

23. Rodgers, J. B., E. M. Riley, G. D. Drummey, and K. J. Isselbacher. Lipid absorption in adrenalectomized rats: the role of altered enzyme activity in the intestinal mucosa. *Gastroenterology* **53:** 547–556, 1967.

24. Stahlgren, L. Presented Before Philadelphia G.I. Research Forum, May 1968.

25. Spencer, R. P., H. Stern, and W. R. Thayer, Jr. Studies on the dynamics of pepsinogen distribution. *Yale J. Biol. Med.* **38:** 417–430, 1965–66.

26. Unger, R. H., H. Ketterer, J. Dupré, and A. M. Eisentraut. The effects of secretin, pancreozymin and gastrin on insulin and glucagon secretion in anesthetized dogs. *J. Clin. Invest.* **46:** 630–645, 1967.

27. Watten, R. H., F. M. Morgan, Y. N. Songkhla, B. Vanikiati, and R. A. Phillips. Water and electrolytes studies in cholera. *J. Clin Invest.* **38:** 1879–1889, 1959.

28. Wells, H. Functional and pharmacological studies on the regulation of salivary gland growth. In: *Secretory Mechanism of the Salivary Glands*. Edited by L. H. and C. A. Schneyer. New York: Academic Press, 1967, pp. 178–190.

29. Wiernik, G., R. G. Shorter, and B. Creamer. The arrest of intestinal epithelial "turnover" by the use of x-irradiation. *Gut* **3:** 26–31, 1962.

Additional Reading

Davenport, H. W. *Physiology of the Digestive Tract* (2nd ed.). Chicago: Year Book Medical Publishers, 1966.

Glass, G. B. J. *Introduction to Gastrointestinal Physiology*. Englewood Cliffs, N.J.: Prentice-Hall, 1968.

Magee, D. F. *Gastro-intestinal Physiology*. Springfield, Ill.: Charles C Thomas, 1962.

Spencer, R. P. *The Intestinal Tract*. Springfield, Ill.: Charles C Thomas, 1960.

Texter, E. C., Jr., C-C Chou, H. C. Laureta, and G. R. Vantrappen. *Physiology of the Gastrointestinal Tract*. St. Louis: C. V. Mosby Co., 1968.

2

Secretion

SECRETION can be characterized in reference to groups of cells arranged in such a fashion that two opposite surfaces of the cells are in contact with solutions of different composition. Constituents of one solution enter through one surface, and constituents of the second leave through the other surface under conditions requiring energy for the process. In the case of the digestive enzymes, the raw materials for enzyme synthesis enter at one surface, and the synthesized enzymes leave at the opposite. In intact secretory glands of the gastrointestinal tract it is often not possible to adhere to such strict criteria. The contents of the lumina of digestive glands are often referred to as secretion even though the concentration of some of the constituents is similar to that in extracellular fluid. It is sometimes not possible to distinguish between movement through cells and between cells. Lowenstein and his associates (3) have presented evidence from electrophysiologic techniques that the movement of electrolytes between cells in the salivary glands is relatively free but that movement across the luminal surface is impeded.

The movement of ions against an electrochemical gradient is defined as active transport. This can be specified more easily in an in vitro system where the potential difference across the membrane and the difference in concentrations between the solutions on either side of the membrane are known. Curran (2) has further refined this definition to exclude transport where the energy is derived by coupling to other active processes. The movement of ions in many of the digestive glands has been defined in these terms.

One of the goals of gastrointestinal physiology is to relate structure to function. In the case of the digestive glands the demonstration of intracellular granules with particular staining techniques made it possible for light microscopy to correlate the disappearance of these granules with the appearance of specific digestive properties in the secretion from the gland. Histochemical techniques have further extended this type of analysis. With the availability of the greatly increased magnification of the electron microscope, many of these experiments have been repeated in order to define secretion in terms of ultrastructure. Autoradiography has made it possible to follow the incorporation of raw materials into the secretory granules and to follow their movement into the lumen of the gland.

As the chemical structure of digestive enzymes becomes known, analytical techniques improve and immunologic techniques may be used to identify the location of physiologically active molecules within the cells. Some substances such as "mucus" still resist quantitative analysis because of their great chemical complexity and heterogeneity.

The structural correlates of the movement of water and electrolytes are still unknown. Electron microscopy has shown marked differences between parietal cells of the stomach at rest and under stimulation, but it is still not possible to examine the structure of ducts of the digestive glands and predict the nature of ion movement across cell surfaces.

Electron microscopists have been impressed by the appearance of protrusion of cytoplasm from cells lining the digestive gland ducts which appear to engulf particulate material and pass it inward to the cell. This is called pinocytosis. Unfortunately, observing this phenomenon under the microscope does not provide quantitative data on its importance in the movement of specific substances.

Although cells have the capacity for secretion, under normal circumstances in vivo, secretion is usually under the control of nervous or hormonal mechanisms or a combination of both. Nervous control lies within the autonomic nervous system. As formulated by Langley, this system consisted of the sympathetic chains and ganglia and the parasympathetic cranial and sacral efferent neurons. Unfortunately this classification leaves no room for afferent neurons or the limbic system in the brain, which is obviously concerned with autonomic function, or the afferent fibers that clearly make contact with the autonomic efferent neurons. Perhaps *visceral nervous system* should be the term used for this purpose (4). To further compound the difficulties in relating structure to function, the precise relationship of nerve endings to secretory or smooth muscle cells is unknown, and the pathways of sympathetic and parasympathetic nerve fibers once they reach the myenteric plexuses are also obscure. Only in the case of the salivary glands is there good evidence that single secretory cells are supplied by both cholinergic and adrenergic neurons.

The demonstration by Bayliss and Starling that a blood-borne stimulus prepared from an extract of intestinal mucosa could stimulate pancreatic secretion in the absence of nervous connections was the foundation of endocrinology. Some of the digestive glands seem to be predominantly under hormonal control, while others are primarily under the influence of the nervous system. Recently abundant evidence has appeared closely linking nervous and humoral factors. The effects of nervous stimulation may be weakened by removing the source of a hormone, and hormonal stimulation may be much less effective in the absence of cholinergic mechanisms.

Nervous control must be considered at the level of the digestive tube or gland itself. In many instances this mechanism can function in the absence of extrinsic nervous factors. However, under normal circumstances, it is apparent that extrinsic nerves do exert an influence on function and that this in turn is organized at various levels within the central nervous system.

The composition of the secretions of the digestive glands fall into three general categories: (1) proteins, particularly those constituting the digestive enzymes; (2) mucopolysaccharides, as in mucus; and (3) solutions of water and electrolytes, as in hydrochloric acid and bicarbonate. Through the use of radioactively labeled amino acids, the qualitative aspects of the formation of digestive enzymes has been at least partially solved. They can be traced from the microsomes of the endoplasmic reticulum into the Golgi apparatus and on through what appears to be a system of tubules within the cytoplasm to the cell surface bordering on the lumen. The site of formation of the protein is in the microsomes. The zymogen molecule is inactive and requires splitting off a fragment before it acquires the ability to attack the appropriate substrate.

Our understanding of the formation of mucus is less complete. Although the structural basis for the secretion of mucus from goblet cells has been established, the chemical nature is more complex. Although mucus-secreting cells look alike under the microscope, studies with isotopically labeled sulfur show that they incorporate this element to varying degrees in different portions of the digestive tract; and indeed in different species the same portion may or may not incorporate sulfur. The fundamental problem is the precise chemical composition of mucus. Present techniques usually characterize only the sugar moiety, such as glucosamine, or one of the many constituents, such as neuraminic (or sialic) acid.

The absence of a structural basis for the secretion of water and electrolytes has already been noted. Much effort has been expended on the general problem of movement across membranes. The most popular hypothesis has involved a hypothetical carrier molecule which "ferries" the molecule to be transported across the membrane. After releasing its cargo it presumably shuttles back to become available for another load. Unfortunately nothing is known of its chemical structure. The definition of the phenomenon of active transport grows more rigorous. Movement must occur in the absence of a favorable concentration or electrical gradient. In order to satisfy these criteria, measurements must be made of the movement of the ion in question with simultaneous recording of concentration and potential difference. Contributing factors such as solvent drag and facilitated diffusion must be considered. In spite of these demands the ability of the stomach to secrete HCl at a concentration of approximately 170 mEq/L, and the pancreas to secrete bicarbonate at 140 mEq/L, remains remarkable and worthy of further study.

In many instances the ionic concentration of intestinal secretions approaches that of interstitial fluid, suggesting equilibrium with that body fluid compartment. Indeed, with the possible exception of saliva, the total osmotic activity of secretions is usually that of extracellular fluid. Correlating these changes with structure and noting the comparison with the renal tubule, it is tempting to suggest that, in the compound acinar gland, the primary secretion elaborated in the acini is modified as it passes through the ducts by exchanges across the ductal epithelium. Indirect evidence for this includes a relationship between flow and composition, stop-flow studies, and the effects of stimulants which are presumed to act only on specific cell groups. However, direct evidence by micropuncture is available only in the salivary glands, where proximal fluid has shown isotonicity in comparison to hypotonic concentrations in the terminal ducts.

After defining the cellular basis for secretion, there remains the problem of its control in the intact organism. Although digestive glands appear to secrete continuously in some species, in many others there is little or no "basal" secretion. The problem of defining basal conditions is obviously of critical importance. If digestive secretions occur intermittently, then what are the stimuli responsible for evoking secretion? Pavlov and his students placed the major responsibility for the control of secretion upon the nervous system and principally the central nervous system. They used the techniques of teasing with food and sham feeding to demonstrate that the CNS via the vagi was of great importance in the control of secretion. Then in 1902, Bayliss and Starling opened a new avenue of approach by the demonstration that a chemical messenger, or *hormone,* as they called it, secretin, had the capacity to profoundly alter pancreatic secretion independently of nervous factors. While the nervous system retained its importance in the control of salivary and gastric secretion, the control of pancreatic and biliary secretion appeared to be primarily independent of the nervous system. More recently, with the characterization of gastrin by Gregory and his associates, it seems likely that the relationship between nervous and hormonal control is closer than had been appreciated. Current evidence suggests that most of the effects of vagal stimulation on the digestive glands can be explained by the release of gastrin from the pyloric antrum (5). There remain the major problems of what are the signals both within and without the intestinal canal that elicit the secretory response and how are they integrated within the cerebral cortex, the autonomic nervous system, and the intestinal tract itself. There are clues from other fields. The specific chemical reactions affected by corticotropin in the adrenal cortex are being identified. Acetylcholine is the chemical mediator at certain myoneural junctions. Behavior, including learning, can be related to chemical changes within the brain. The control of body temperature and respiration is now being approached in terms of specific cell receptors responding to deviations from a set point such as body temperature and pCO_2. These represent encouraging signs for our future understanding of the neurohumoral control of the secretion of the digestive glands.

References

1. Bayliss, L. E. *Principles of General Physiology*, Vol. 2. London: Longmans, Green, 1960, pp. 362–405.
2. Curran, P. F. Coupling between transport processes in the intestine. *Physiologist* 11: 3–23, 1968.
3. Lowenstein, W. R., S. J. Socolar, S. Higashino, Y. Kanno, and N. Davidson. Intercellular communication: renal, urinary bladder sensory and salivary gland cells. *Science* 149: 295–298, 1965.
4. Monnier, M. *Functions of the Nervous System*, Vol. 1. New York: Elsevier Publishing Co., 1968, p. 92.
5. Grossman, M. I. (ed.). *Gastrin*. Berkeley and Los Angeles: University of California Press, 1966.

Salivary Secretion

THE SALIVARY GLANDS offer a number of advantages to the student of secretion; they are relatively accessible, there is a well-developed acinus-ductal system, and they are under the control of the autonomic nervous system. Salivary ducts were the first to be subjected to successful micropuncture. The major disadvantage is the analytical problem in quantitating mucus, one of the important constituents of saliva.

Structural Basis for the Control of Saliva

The acinar cells of the salivary glands can be divided into three categories based upon histochemistry and light and electron microscopy (13). Serous cells contain small refractile granules and variable amounts of mucopolysaccharides. They are probably the source of amylase. For this reason serous granules have been referred to as zymogen granules, but there is no evidence that the amylase exists in an inactive form. Mucous cells contain droplets of mucinogen and acid mucopolysaccharides. A third group shares characteristics of both, containing acidic and neutral mucopolysaccharides, and are known as seromucous cells.

The individual salivary acinus may be composed of a mixture of cell types or largely a single variety. The parotid is essentially a purely serous gland and the sublingual a mucous gland, while the submaxillary is mixed. The serous cells in the acini of the submaxillary gland lie at the opposite pole of the acinus from the duct, forming a crescent or demilune. They usually com-

16

municate with a lumen via a system of secretory capillaries which pass between the mucous cells.

The structure of the salivary ducts varies with species of animals. Figure 3-1 shows the structure of the ducts of the major salivary glands in man. The epithelium of the intercalated ducts is low, with the nuclei filling much of the cytoplasm. The striated ducts take their name from the appearance of basal striations, which on electron microscopy are the result of extensive infolding of the basal cell membrane around mitochondria. The latter are arranged in a series of parallel columns. These cells are of great interest in the secretion of electrolytes. They have a counterpart in the kidney tubule.

The blood supply of the salivary glands travels to the ducts where it breaks up into a rich plexus around the ducts. Branches to the alveoli come off near the ends of the intralobular ducts and form a plexus which is much less extensive than that around the ducts.

For the most part, nerve fibers can be traced into the stroma (parasympathetic?) or in association with blood vessels (sympathetic). Only in the case of the acinar cells of the parotid and sublingual have nerve endings been identified in close approximation to the secretory cells. Gomez (7) found two nerve fibers running together in the perialveolar plexus of human lingual acini and postulated that they represented parasympathetic and sympathetic fibers.

Stimulation of salivary secretion results in degranulation of the secretory

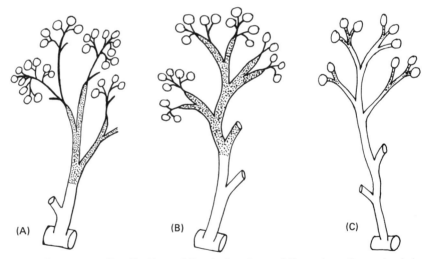

FIGURE 3-1.   Ramifications of the duct systems of the major salivary glands in the human. A: parotid; B: submaxillary; C: sublingual. *Solid black:* intercalated ducts; *stippled:* striated ducts; *unshaded:* interlobular and interlobar ducts. (From C. R. Leeson, Structure of salivary glands. In: *Handbook of Physiology*, Section 6: Alimentary Tract. Vol. 2: Secretion. Edited by C. F. Code. Washington, D.C.: American Physiological Society, 1967, pp. 463–495.)

cells (24). Unlike the pancreas there is no direct spatial relationship between the Golgi apparatus and newly formed granules. The mucous cells discharge their granules without disrupting the luminal membrane, in contrast to the goblet cells of the intestine.

Water and Electrolyte Secretion

The composition of saliva obtained from individual glands will vary with the rate of secretion, the nature of the stimulus, and the species of animal. Furthermore there are striking but unexplained differences in the composition of saliva from different glands secreted in response to the same stimulus (21). As a result, there is no simple answer to the question, what is the composition of saliva? In general, sodium and potassium are the principal cations, and bicarbonate and chloride the main anions. Perhaps the best recalled unusual characteristic of saliva is that in some species, including man, it may be hypotonic with respect to extracellular fluid, especially at low rates of flow.

Figure 3-2 shows the relationship between flow and composition of saliva from the human parotid gland. The pH of human mixed saliva is usually slightly acidic (6,7). The difference between the ionic composition of parotid saliva and plasma is shown also in Figure 3-2.

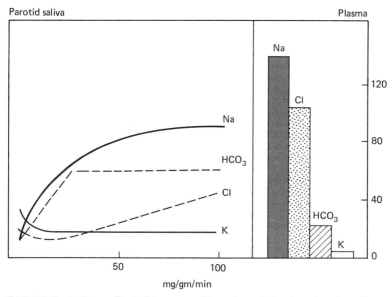

FIGURE 3-2.   Electrolyte composition of parotid saliva at various flow rates. Abscissa secretory rate in mg/gm of saliva per gland per minute. Ordinate concentration in milliequivalents/liter.   From F. Bro-Rasmussen, S. Killman, and J. H. Thaysen. *Acta Physiol. Scand.* **37:** 97, 1956.)

As a first approach to the origin of the water and electrolyte in salivary secretion, one might attempt to distinguish between the acini and ducts as a source. Unfortunately the evidence is conflicting. Micropuncture studies in the submaxillary gland of rat show that the sodium and chloride concentrations of saliva at the end of the intercalated ducts resemble closely that of an ultrafiltrate of plasma (32). No data on bicarbonate concentrations were available and micropuncture of the acinus has not been accomplished. In many species the ducts develop before the acini. Such ducts are capable of forming saliva of similar electrolyte composition. Junqueira makes the interesting comment that only in species with striated ducts does the development of ducts precede that of acini (10). When the compositions of saliva at different levels of the ductal system were compared in rat submaxillary gland, a more complex series of events emerged. During passage through the striated ducts there was a significant reabsorption of sodium and a secretion of potassium even at high flow rates. In the more distal ducts reequilibration with plasma occurred if flow was slow enough. Finally, in the main duct, reabsorption of sodium and secretion of potassium occurred again if contact time permitted.

Yoshimura has also provided evidence for ductal secretion using the submaxillary gland of the dog perfused with Locke's solution (31). He attempted to collect postacinar secretion by puncture. Similar conclusions were drawn from the loss of the usual relation of flow to composition after injecting mercuric chloride retrograde into the salivary ducts.

In contrast, the role of the acini is supported by indirect evidence, largely from electrophysiologic studies. Lundberg, using intracellular electrodes, identified acinar cells in the cat sublingual gland with resting membrane potentials of -22 mv (15). If the electrode were advanced into the lumen the potential with respect to the surface of the gland fell to no more than a few millivolts. However, if the chorda tympani nerve were stimulated with repetitive electrical shocks, the intracellular potential fell another 25 to 40 mv. If the electrode were again pushed into the lumen, the same degree of hyperpolarization was seen. Lundberg interpreted these results to indicate that the apical cell membrane did not respond to stimulation while the basal membrane became hyperpolarized. At the same time the conductance of the basal membrane increased, and he concluded that the most likely explanation was an active transport of chloride into the cell. These results would explain the formation of acinar secretion as secondary to the active transport of chloride (2).

The correlation between electrophysiologic events and secretion has not been clear in the experience of other workers. Petersen and his colleagues, using a perfused cat submaxillary gland, found that chloride could be replaced by sulfate with maintenance of a secretory potential but without secretion (17). Yoshimura invoked pinocytosis to account for acinar secretion (31). Therefore the contribution of the acini to electrolyte secretion remains uncertain.

Langley and Brown used stop-flow techniques, which had been successful in the kidney, to identify transport sites in the parotid gland (12). After a period of occlusion, saliva was collected in serial small fractions. The ion to be studied was injected intraarterially as an isotope. The longer the delay before the radioactivity appeared, the more proximal the transport site in the duct. They found that iodide entered proximally and calcium distally. Sodium and chloride concentrations fell during occlusion while potassium, calcium, iodide, and phosphate concentrations rose. Since water also left the duct, these results are difficult to interpret. But they do show that transfer does occur across the epithelium of the ducts.

The relatively high concentration of bicarbonate in human parotid saliva (60 mM) raises questions as to its source. That the plasma bicarbonate contributes significantly is evident from isotope studies. Unfortunately we cannot distinguish between transport into the cells as CO_2 or bicarbonate. Endogenous CO_2 production by the cells can also contribute to salivary bicarbonate but probably to a minor extent (21).

Salivary Proteins and Mucin

Saliva contains variable amounts of protein. The best-studied protein is salivary amylase (5). It has a molecular weight of about 50,000. Crystalline salivary amylase is a mixture of at least 7 proteins. It appears that salivary amylase exists as a series of isoenzymes. Amylase is probably released from ribosomes in an active form (22). In the rat about 50 per cent of the amylase is present in secretory granules, and 30 to 40 per cent of protein in the granules is amylase. Secretory granules constitute about one third of the cell protein. Amylase appears first in the ribosomes, then in the cell supernatant, and finally in the secretory granules. With extrusion of amylase from the cell the membrane of the secretory granule remains in the cell. During the first three hours of incubation of slices of rat parotid, the secreted amylase is derived entirely from that in secretory granules. Later the cell supernatant contributes.

Another interesting salivary protein is the immunoglobulin IgA. In contrast to its form in serum, it is coupled to a secretory piece or beta globulin which is secreted by the salivary epithelium (27).

Radioactively labeled amino acids injected into the circulation of dogs appear in the saliva both as free amino acids and incorporated into proteins (8). The salivary-plasma ratios for individual amino acids vary widely without apparent explanation.

Salivary glycoproteins are a complex group of substances (5). They include blood group substances and various mucins. The structure of only a few of the latter has been identified. Figure 3-3 shows a portion of the molecule of ovine submaxillary gland protein. Note the polypeptide core with the polysaccharides attached.

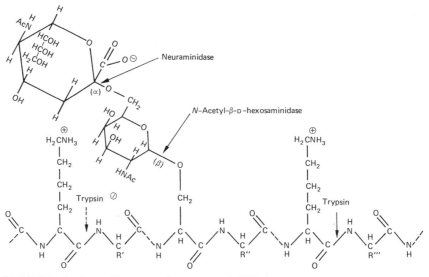

FIGURE 3-3.   Diagrammatic segment of OSM showing the structure of the carbohydrate group, its glycosidic linkage to a seryl residue, the enzymes which cleave the glycosidic linkages involving the two sugar components, and a trypsin-susceptible and a trypsin-resistant peptide bond. (Reproduced from A. Gottschalk, (ed.). *Glycoproteins: Their Composition, Structure and Function.* Amsterdam: Elsevier, 1966, p. 434.)

Horowitz, in an extensive review of salivary mucins, classifies them into two major categories: mucopolysaccharides and glycoproteins (9). Mucopolysaccharides are large molecules made up of chains of amino sugars. They may be further divided into neutral and acid mucopolysaccharides. The latter contain a uronic acid or sulfate ester or both groupings. Glycoproteins are macromolecules containing oligosaccharides linked to a protein core. They may be subclassified as neutral, acid, or mixed, depending upon the groupings at the ends of the oligosaccharides. Finally, mucopolysaccharides can interact with proteins to form complexes by salt linkages or by covalent bonds. Examples are shown in the following listing:

Glycoproteins	Synonyms	Functional Significance
Neutral	Fucomucins	Blood group substance A
Acid	Sialomucins	Bovine submaxillary mucin
Mixed		Blood group substance Lewis

At present it is not possible to correlate the viscous properties of saliva with the molecular structure of any known mucopolysaccharide or glycoprotein. Similarly, little is known of the sequence of events in the synthesis of these substances. Race and Sanger (18) suggested that the ABH blood group substances and the Lewis substance are derived from a common precursor.

The epithelial cells of individuals secreting the ABH substances direct nearly all the precursor substance into ABH, while nonsecretors of ABH have an abundance of precursor available for the synthesis of Lewis substance. There are striking differences in the composition of parotid and submaxillary mucins as determined by the present rather crude methods.

Most investigators have found traces of plasma proteins in saliva. However, how they enter saliva is unknown. Many studies are done on salivary tissue rather than saliva which would account for some differences between large molecules in saliva and those in the tissues.

The Metabolism of Salivary Secretion

It is a standard laboratory experiment to inject pilocarpine intravenously into a cat and show that the submaxillary gland will secrete against a pressure much higher than the mean arterial pressure and thereby to exclude simple filtration as a mechanism for the formation of saliva. Salivary glands are characterized by a high rate of oxygen consumption, but when the glands are stimulated, blood flow increases to an even greater degree, so that the oxygen supply is not limited (16). The additional work required to produce a hypotonic saliva represents only a small fraction of the energy available.

In many epithelia, a sodium-potassium ATPase plays an important role in membrane transport. Schwartz and Moore have achieved partial purification of such an enzyme from the parotid of dog (23). This enzyme could play an important role in the transport of sodium out of the lumen in the striated ducts.

Glucose appears to be the preferred substrate for the support of stimulated salivary secretion and the Embden-Meyerhof glycolytic pathway was more important than the pentose phosphate pathway in the rat submaxillary gland in vitro (16). The relationship between extrusion and enzyme synthesis in the salivary glands is unclear.

The Control of Salivary Secretion

Cellular control mechanisms have already been mentioned in the introduction. In most instances salivary glands deprived of an extrinsic nervous supply cease to secrete. The exceptions are the sublingual gland of cat, dog, and rat; the submaxillary gland of rabbit; and the parotid of ruminants (16). These exceptions provide examples of secretory cells that resemble certain smooth muscle cells in their capacity to exhibit unstimulated activity. This represents "spontaneous" secretion. Man, on the other hand, shows "continuous secretion" during the day, but virtually ceases secretion during sleep. That continuous secretion is dependent upon impulses reaching the glands via the chorda tympani nerve is suggested by cessation of secretion when the nerve has been cut.

The extrinsic control of salivary secretion must be related to the nervous system, the endocrine glands, and the circulation. In most experiments on the control of salivation, saliva was collected from the main duct so that the site of action of the control mechanism was unknown. Yoshimura (31) has provided some interesting evidence that parasympathetic stimulation of salivary secretion in the dog submaxillary gland is dependent upon a nervous reflex to the ducts. Using a perfused gland, he showed that secretion was modified in response to changes in osmolarity of the blood to the brain and that the efferent limb of the reflex reached the ductal cells via cholinergic fibers in the chorda tympani, vagus, and hypoglossal nerves. The striated ducts responded by increasing the transport of sodium.

In general the parasympathetic supply to the salivary glands exerts the dominant nervous control of salivary secretion. Figure 3-4 shows the pathways from the brain. In the rat, parasympathectomy results in a marked fall in the amount of amylase in the parotid gland and in its concentration in parotid secretion. The size of the cells of the acini and striated ducts is reduced (20).

The effects of the sympathetic division of the autonomic nervous system on the salivary glands are more difficult to define, since in addition to an effect on the secretory cells, sympathetic stimulation may produce significant vaso-constriction and contraction of the myoepitheial cells with expression of fluid from the contents of the ducts. However, most investigators believe that sympathetic nerves do carry secretory fibers to the salivary glands and, in the case of the submaxillary glands, play a significant role in secretion particularly on the acinar cells.

There has been much speculation over the innervation of these mixed glands. Based upon degranulation after stimulation, investigators in the past suggested that the serous cells were supplied by the parasympathetic and the mucous cells by the sympathetic. Histologic techniques have failed to help, but intracellular potential recordings indicate changes in the same cell upon stimulation of both parasympathetic and sympathetic nerves (15).

Reflex control of salivary secretion attained almost legendary status through the experiments of Pavlov on conditioned reflexes. These result from the association of normally ineffective stimuli (ringing a bell) with uniformally effective stimuli (feeding). After a time the latter can be omitted while the response (salivation) continues. Considering Pavlov's interest in the stomach it is interesting that he did so little with conditioning of gastric secretion. Early studies centered on the question of what parts of the central nervous system were involved. It now seems clear that the cerebral cortex is not required.

Unconditioned reflexes play an important part in the control of salivary secretion. Mechanoreceptors and chemoreceptors in the nose and mouth re-spond to appropriate stimuli and elicit secretion via the salivary nuclei in

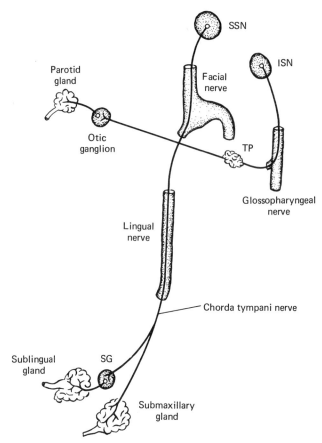

FIGURE 3-4. Diagram of the parasympathetic nerve supply of the salivary glands. SSN: superior salivatory nucleus; ISN: inferior salivatory nucleus; SG: submaxillary ganglion; TP: tympanic plexus. (From N. C. Hightower. Salivary secretion. In: *Physiological Basis of Medical Practice*, 8th ed. Edited by C. H. Best and N. B. Taylor. © 1966, The Williams & Wilkins Co., Baltimore, Md. 21202, U.S.A.)

the medulla. Unfortunately, little is known of the language in these afferents. The frequency of impulses which indicates properties of the excitant elsewhere does not serve that function for smell and taste. In man, the electrolyte and protein content of saliva seems to depend upon flow independent of the nature of the stimulation (3).

The cerebral cortex and afferent fibers in the sciatic nerve share similar efferent parasympathetic and sympathetic pathways to the submaxillary glands in cats (28). Figure 3-5 shows these pathways. The center for efferent control of salivation lies in the pons and medulla, as shown in Figure 3-6. Note their proximity to centers for the control of respiration and vasomotion. Reflex salivation from the submaxillary gland can be obtained as long as the level

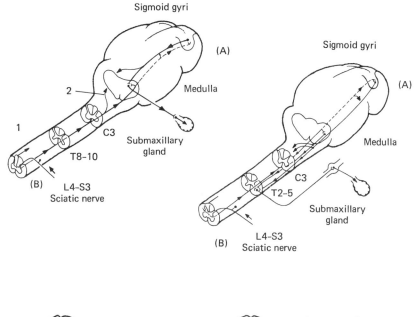

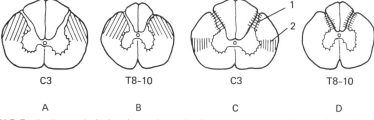

FIGURE 3-5. *Left drawing:* schematic diagram showing pathways for activation of the submandibular gland via its parasympathetic innervation (A): from Loci on the sigmoid gyri of the frontal lobes and (B): from the central end of the sciatic nerve. The afferent pathway from the sciatic crosses at spinal (1) and supraspinal (2) levels and affects the superior salivary nucleus in the medulla. The descending corticofugal pathway is both crossed and uncrossed. Possible activation of this descending pathway at cortical, hypo-thalamic, and other levels by ascending fibers above the medulla is indicated (dotted lines). *Four bottom drawings:* localization in the cord of an afferent pathway from the sciatic nerve mediating submandibular salivary responses via parasympathetic or sympa-thetic innervation (A) at C_3 and (B) at T8–10. Bilateral section of the dorsal horn and Lissauer's tract at the cervical (C) or thoracic (D) levels does not interrupt the afferent tract. The efferent sympathetic path from both cortex and sciatic lies in the cervical cord at the junction of the dorsal and ventral half of the lateral funiculus (C). *Right drawing:* Diagrammatic scheme for activation of the submandibular gland via its sympathetic inner-vation. (A): from the frontal lobe and (B): from the central end of the sciatic nerve. Spinal crossing of the afferent pathway and its possible direct effect on preganglionic sympa-thetic nerons as well as its medullary connections are shown. As in the case of the para-sympathetic activation of the gland, the descending corticofugal path is crossed and un-crossed. Hypothesized afferent fibers above the medullary level are indicated (dotted lines). (From A. G. Velo, and E. C. Hoff. *Amer. J. Physiol.* **200:** 46–50, 1961.)

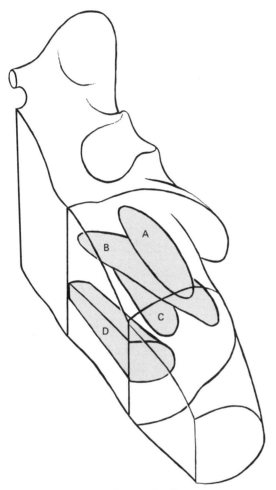

FIGURE 3-6.   Perspective illustration of anatomical relationships within the medulla of responsive regions for A: spasmodic respiratory movement; B: salivation; C: vomiting; and D: forced inspiration. (From Borison and S. C. Wang. *J. Neurophysiol.* **12:** 311, 1949.)

of section is rostral to the facial nucleus (29). Points for stimulation of the parotid lie 1 to 2 mm caudal to those for the submaxillary in the cat. Both glands respond to ipsilateral stimulation, whereas the contralateral response is weak. The level of activity in these nuclei is thought to be under the control of the cerebral cortex, hypothalamus, and amygdala, which serves to integrate feeding patterns with salivation.

There is no hormone that exerts a control over normal functioning of salivary secretion, with the exception of epinephrine. In ruminants the salivary glands play a more important role in fluid balance, and parotid secretion is exquisitely sensitive to aldosterone, responding with a decreased sodium-potassium ratio to as little as 4 units of intravenous aldosterone per hour. In man with abnormally elevated levels of aldosterone in the circulation, the ratio of sodium to potassium in saliva falls, owing largely to a decrease in the concentration of sodium. This must be interpreted with regard to flow, since sodium concentrations rise with increasing flow. In the toad bladder, Edelman and his associates (4) suggested that aldosterone entered secretory cells and reached the nucleus when it acted upon DNA to lead to the formation of messenger RNA. The latter directed protein synthesis in the cytoplasm, resulting in a change in sodium transport across the cell membrane. Junqueira writes that the inhibitory action of vasopressin on salivary flow is unaffected by actinomycin D or puromycin and therefore does not share this mechanism of control (10).

In experimental animals hypophysectomy results in loss of weight and decreased size of the acinar cells of the parotid. The epithelium of the ducts was reduced in height (1). There are fewer secretory granules and decreased amylase content. The gland can be restored to normal by somatotropin, thyroxin, and corticosterone. Effects on the submaxillary gland were less pronounced and the sublingual was unaffected. Baker and his associates consider these to be nonspecific effects on protein synthesis (1).

The role of blood supply to salivary glands in the control of salivary secretion has already been mentioned. Earlier investigators had explained vasodilation coincident with secretion as resulting from stimulation of parasympathetic vasodilator fibers. Hilton and Lewis isolated a polypeptide, bradykinin, with vasodilator properties. They suggested that stimuli to secretion lead to release of an enzyme that acts on a plasma globulin to form bradykinin. Originally they proposed that this might be a general mechanism for vasodilation but more recently Lewis has restricted its role (14). Schachter has assembled evidence that cholinergic vasodilator fibers are responsible for most of the effects on the circulation of the salivary glands coincident with secretion (19). Vasoconstriction in response to sympathetic stimulation can reduce salivary flow, particularly at high rates of secretion.

Growth and Adaptation of Salivary Glands

The ability of the digestive glands to modify their secretion in response to changes in diet was a major interest of Pavlov and his school. Squires found that subjects on a high-carbohydrate diet had twice the concentration of salivary amylase of subjects on a high-protein diet (26). There are a number of experimental situations that produce hypertrophy, hyperplasia, or atrophy of salivary glands and provide clues for control mechanisms (30). Liquid diets in rats lead to a reduction in the size of salivary acinar cells. On the other hand, a calorically inert bulk diet increased the size of acinar cells. Presumably sensory receptors initiate impulses which reach the CNS and lead to efferent activity in the parasympathetics. Cutting the parasympathetic nerves prevents the change in cell size. Removal of the lower central incisors also produces enlarged acinar cells, but this effect is dependent upon sympathetic as well as parasympathetic nerves. The drug isoproterenol, which acts on beta receptors, produces hypertrophy and hyperplasia of the acinar cells (25). Coincidentally, the RNA content of the gland and RNA synthesis increases.

Function of the Salivary Glands in Man

Salivary secretion in man has three major functions; it protects the teeth against decay, it participates in the control of water intake, and it begins the digestive process. Loss of salivation accelerates dental caries. A dry mouth increases water intake, and salivary amylase begins the digestion of starch.

Pathophysiology

The major significance of disturbances in salivary physiology comes from the use of drugs that mimic or inhibit the actions of the autonomic nervous system. Anticholinergic, antisecretory, or antispasmodic agents that interfere with the action of acetylcholine at the neurosecretory or myoneural junction also lead to a dry mouth. In some instances this may be a limiting factor in the use of the drug. However, it also serves as a simple clinical guide in the use of the agent. Doses that produce dry mouth may be assumed to usually reduce gastric secretion in patients with peptic ulcer.

Summary

Salivary secretion is composed of water, electrolytes, proteins, and glycoproteins. The most likely hypothesis for the formation of the inorganic portion of saliva is that the acini form an ultrafiltrate of the plasma which is modified by the removal of sodium and addition of bicarbonate in the ducts. All three transport steps presumably involve energy-requiring processes. Proteins and glycoproteins are added by extrusion from secretory granules in the acinar cells. Control of salivary secretion resides largely with the autonomic nervous system, particularly the parasympathetic division. Effects on the cell may involve genetic control of protein synthesis or direct effects on cell membranes. The clinical importance of salivary secretion lies in its susceptibility to the action of autonomic stimulating and blocking drugs.

References

1. Baker, B. L., H. W. Clapp, Jr., and J. A. Light. Hormonal influences on cytology and physiology of salivary glands. In: *Salivary Glands and Their Secretions.* Edited by L. M. Sreebny and J. Meyer. New York: The Macmillan Co., 1964, pp. 63–82.

2. Burgen, A. S. V. Membrane potentials and the secretory activity of acinar cells. In: *The Secretory Mechanisms of Salivary Glands.* Edited by L. H. and C. A. Schneyer. New York: Academic Press, 1967, pp. 3–10.

3. Dawes, C., and G. N. Jenkins. The effects of different stimuli on the composition of saliva in man. *J. Physiol., London* **170:** 86–100, 1964.

4. Edelman, I. S., R. Bogoroch, and G. A. Porter. On the mechanism of action of aldosterone on sodium transport: the role of protein synthesis. *Proc. Nat. Acad. Sci. USA* **50:** 1169–1176, 1963.

5. Ellison, S. A. Proteins and glycoproteins of saliva. In: *Handbook of Physiology.* Section 6: Alimentary Tract. Vol. 2: Secretion. Edited by C. F. Code. Washington, D.C.: American Physiological Society, 1967, pp. 531–559.

6. Emmelin, N. Secretion from denervated salivary glands. In: *The Secretory Mechanisms of Salivary Glands.* Edited by L. H. and C. A. Schneyer. New York: Academic Press, 1967, pp. 127–141.

7. Gomez, H. The innervation of lingual salivary glands. *Anat. Rec.* **139:** 69–80, 1961.

8. Hanson, R. W., O. L. Catanzaro, and R. H. Lindsay. Secretion of amino acids in dog parotid saliva. *Am. J. Physiol.* **214:** 1068–1073, 1968.

9. Horowitz, M. L. Mucopolysaccharides and glycoproteins of the alimentary tract. In: *Handbook of Physiology.* Section 6: Alimentary Tract. Vol. 2: Secretion. Edited by C. F. Code. Washington, D.C.: American Physiological Society, 1967, pp. 1063–1085.

10. Junqueira, L. C. U. Control of cell secretion. In: *The Secretory Mechanisms of Salivary Glands.* Edited by L. H. and C. A. Schneyer. New York: Academic Press, 1967, pp. 286–302.

11. Lamberts, B. L., and T. S. Meyer. Amylolytic fractions of salivary secretion. In: *The Secretory Mechanisms of Salivary Glands.* Edited by L. H. and C. A. Schneyer. New York: Academic Press, 1967, pp. 313–325.

12. Langley, L. L., and R. S. Brown. Stop-flow analysis of ionic transfer in the dog parotid gland. *Am. J. Physiol.* **199:** 59–62, 1960.

13. Leeson, C. R. Structure of salivary glands. In: *Handbook of Physiology.* Section 6: Alimentary Tract. Vol. 2: Secretion. Edited by C. F. Code. Washington D.C.: American Physiological Society, 1967, pp. 463–495.

14. Lewis, G. P. The role of plasma kinins as mediator of functional vasodilation. *Gastroenterology* **52:** 406–413, 1967.

15. Lundberg, A. Electrophysiology of salivary glands. *Physiol. Rev.* **38:** 21–40, 1958.

16. Martin, K. Metabolism of salivary glands. In: *Handbook of Physiology.* Section 6: Alimentary Tract. Vol. 2: Secretion. Edited by C. F. Code. Washington, D.C.: American Physiological Society, 1967, pp. 581–593.

17. Petersen, O. H., J. H. Poulsen, and N. A. Thorn. Secretory potentials, secretory rate and water permeability of the duct system in the cat submandibular gland

during perfusion with calcium-free Locke's solution. *Acta Physiol. Scand.* **71:** 203–210, 1967.

18. Race, R. R., and R. Sanger. *Blood Groups in Man* (3rd. ed.), Oxford: Blackwell Scientific Publications, 1958.

19. Schachter, M., and S. Beilenson. Kallikrein and vasodilation in the submaxillary gland. *Gastroenterology* **52:** 401–405, 1967.

20. Schneyer, C. A., and H. D. Hall. Autonomic regulation of the immature and adult rat parotid gland. In: *The Secretory Mechanisms of Salivary Glands.* Edited by L. H. and C. A. Schneyer. New York: Academic Press, 1967, pp. 155–177.

21. Schneyer, L. H., and C. A. Schneyer. Inorganic composition of saliva. In: *Handbook of Physiology.* Section 6: Alimentary Tract. Vol. 2: Secretion. Edited by C. F. Code. Washington, D.C.: American Physiological Society, 1967, pp. 497–530.

22. Schramm, M. Transport, storage and secretion of amylase in the parotid gland of the rat. In: *Salivary Glands and Their Secretions.* Edited by L. M. Sreebny and J. Meyer. New York: The Macmillan Co., 1964, pp. 315–323.

23. Schwartz, A., and C. A. Moore. Highly active Na$^+$, K$^+$,-ATPase in rat submaxillary gland bearing on salivary secretion. *Am. J. Physiol.* **214:** 1163–1167, 1968.

24. Scott, B. L., and D. C. Pease. Electron microscopy of induced changes in the salivary gland of the rat. In: *Salivary Glands and Their Secretions.* Edited by L. M. Sreebny and J. Meyer. New York: The Macmillan Co., 1964, pp. 13–44.

25. Seifert, G. Experimental sialadenosis by isoproterenol and other agents: histochemistry and electron microscopy. In: *The Secretory Mechanisms of Salivary Glands.* Edited by L. H. and C. A. Schneyer. New York: Academic Press, 1967, pp. 191–208.

26. Squires, B. T. Human salivary amylase secretion in relation to diet. *J. Physiol. London,* **119:** 153–156, 1953.

27. Tomasi, T. B., Jr., E. M. Tan, A. Solomon, and R. Prendergast. Characteristics of an immune system common to certain external secretions. *J. Exp. Med.* **121:** 101–124, 1965.

28. Velo, A. G., and E. C. Hoff. Salivary responses to cortical and sciatic stimulation. *Am. J. Physiol.* **200:** 46–50, 1961.

29. Wang, S. C. Central nervous representation of salivary secretion. In: *Salivary Glands and Their Secretions.* Edited by L. M. Sreebny and J. Meyer. New York: The Macmillan Co., 1964, pp. 145–159.

30. Wells, H. Functional and pharmacological studies on the regulation of salivary gland growth. In: *The Secretory Mechanisms of Salivary Glands.* Edited by L. H. and C. A. Schneyer. New York: Academic Press, 1967, pp. 178–190.

31. Yoshimura, H. Secretory mechanism of saliva and nervous control of its ionic composition. In: *The Secretory Mechanisms of Salivary Glands.* Edited by L. H. and C. A. Schneyer. New York: Academic Press, 1967, pp. 56–74.

32. Young, J. A., E. Fromter, E. Schögel, and K. F. Hamann. Micropuncture and perfusion studies of fluid and electrolyte transport in the rat submaxillary gland. In: *The Secretory Mechanisms of Salivary Glands.* Edited by L. H. and C. A. Schneyer. New York: Academic Press, 1967, pp. 11–31.

Additional Reading

Burgen, A. S. V., and N. G. Emmelin. *Physiology of the Salivary Glands.* London: Edward Arnold (Publishers), Ltd. 1961.

Salivary Glands and Their Secretions, edited by L. M. Sreebny and J. Meyer. New York: The Macmillan Co., 1964.

Secretory Mechanisms of the Salivary Glands, edited by L. H. and C. A. Schneyer. New York: Academic Press, 1967.

CHAPTER

4

Gastric Secretion

THE SECRETORY CAPACITY of the stomach is one of the wonders of the gastro-enterologic world. The stomach has the capacity of varying outputs of hydrochloric acid from zero to over 20 mEq/hour in man. The polypeptide hormone gastrin produced maximal stimulation of acid secretion in man when given subcutaneously in a dose of 2 μg/kg. It is likely that gastrin release and acid production are linked in an autoregulatory mechanism.

Structural Basis of Gastric Secretion (57)

The stomach may be divided grossly into fundus, body, and pyloric antrum, as shown in Figure 4-1. The divisions are arbitrary, but in general the fundic portion lies above the level of the entrance of the esophagus, and the pyloric antrum begins at the level of a prominent fold, the incisura angularis, on the lesser curvature. The term *cardia* refers to the area adjacent to the cardioesophageal junction. In addition to their importance as anatomic landmarks, these divisions are associated with a characteristic type of mucosa. The cardiac area contains cardiac glands, the body is lined with fundic or acid-secreting glands, and the surface of the pyloric antrum is covered with pyloric glands.

The cardiac glands secrete mucus but otherwise have little significance. The fundic glands empty in groups into a short common channel or pit before emptying onto the surface epithelium. Figure 4-2 shows a typical fundic gland. Three major cell types can be distinguished: The most numerous are the chief

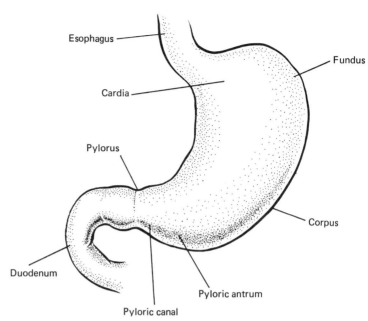

FIGURE 4-1. Anatomy of the stomach. (Adapted from S. Ito. *Anatomic Structure of Gastric Mucosa.* In: *Handbook of Physiology,* Section 6: Alimentary Tract. Vol. 2: Secretion. Edited by C. F. Code. Washington, D.C.: American Physiological Society, 1967. pp. 705–741.)

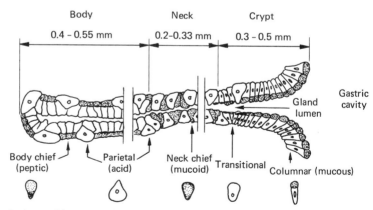

FIGURE 4-2. Diagrammatic representation of the gastric gland tubule (dimensions approximate). (From F. Hollander. *Amer. J. Med.* **13:** 453, 1952.)

cells or zymogen cells, so called because of their secretory granules, thought to represent the inactive or precursor form of pepsin. Concentrated in the midportion of the gland are the parietal or oxyntic cells, thought to be the site of hydrochloric acid formation. They tend to reach the lumen between cells lying on the surface of the gland. Electron microscopy has detected a complex system of intracellular tubules, or canaliculi, lined with microvilli. The formation of HCl is thought to occur at the surface of these tubules. In some species marked changes occur as the resting glands are stimulated to secrete. Figure 4-3 shows the differences in the intracellular tubules when the parietal cells of a frog were stimulated to secrete or subjected to hypoxia. During stimulation the microvilli elongate and the tubules evert, possibly bringing the hypothetical carrier into contact with the luminal contents of the gland. When secretion is inhibited by hypoxia, the microvilli become confluent and possibly convert the tubules into closed vacuoles (86).

One of the best-documented structural relationships in secretion is the direct proportion between the number of parietal cells in the fundic mucosa and the maximal acid secretory output in response to histamine. Figure 4-4 shows this relationship for human stomachs removed from patients with peptic ulcers (13).

The surface epithelial cells line the isthmus of the gland and extend out onto the surface of the fundic mucosa. These cells secrete mucus and contain granules with the staining characteristics of mucopolysaccharides. Not easily distinguished in Figure 4-2 or under the microscope are the mucous neck

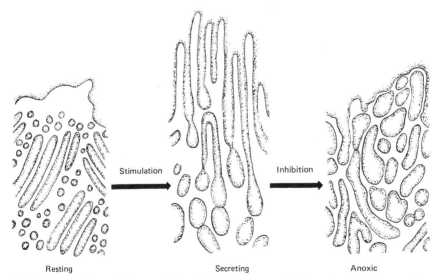

Resting   Secreting   Anoxic

FIGURE 4-3.   Scheme of fine structural changes in the apical cytoplasm of the oxyntic cell during stimulation and inhibition of acid production in the gastric mucosa of the frog. (From A. W. Sedar. *Fed. Proc.* **24:** 1360–1367, 1965.)

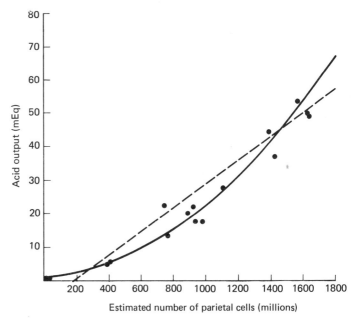

FIGURE 4-4.   Relationship of acid output to parietal cell population of stomach. (From W. I. Card, and I. N. Marks. *Clin. Sci.* **19:** 147, 1960.)

cells. They appear to be intermediate in their characteristics between surface epithelial cells and chief cells. Their granules contain mucus, and the ribosomes are more numerous. There is a better-developed granular endoplasmic reticulum than in the surface epithelial cells. The importance of these cells lies in the indirect evidence that they are the source of regenerating cells for both the glands and the surface epithelium.

The least frequent cell of the fundic glands is the argentaffin or enterochromaffin cell. It is characterized by secretory granules which may represent serotonin (*80*). Argentaffin cells may be subdivided into argyrophil cells which take up the silver stain only after exposure to a reducing agent. The granules are concentrated in the basal portion of the cell and may be secreted into the extracellular space.

The pyloric glands occupy an area equivalent to about one fifth of the gastric mucosa. Surface epithelial cells are present in the isthmus of the glands and in the pits which may occupy one half the total thickness of the epithelium. The glands below the isthmus are lined by cells similar to mucous neck cells. McGuigan has reported that a random selection of these cells demonstrate immunofluorescence with antibodies to gastrin (*64*). Argentaffin cells are present here as well. A few parietal cells may be present.

Immunofluorescence has been used to identify the source of intrinsic factor. In man the cell of origin is the parietal cell (*51*).

Unfortunately a maximal stimulus to pepsin secretion has not been identified to permit a correlation between the number of chief cells and peptic output. Some qualitative differences probably exist between the mucus of surface epithelial cells and the mucous neck cells. The latter incorporate radioactive sulfur in some species.

Cell Renewal in Gastric Mucosa

Tritiated thymidine is incorporated into the DNA of cells undergoing division. This technique has been used to label gastric fundic mucosal cells. Radioautographs showed that epithelial cells migrated from the isthmus to the surface in two to six days (62). Parietal and chief cells showed little synthetic activity and must divide slowly under normal circumstances (63). Amounts of DNA in human gastric content suggest a daily loss of 0.55 million cells a minute (21).

Growth of Gastric Mucosa

In the rat, the growth of the gastric mucosa was determined by body weight rather than by age or sex (19,11b). The parietal cell population varied with the body weight raised to the power 0.9. A strong positive correlation existed between total parietal cell population and the volume of the fundic mucosa ($r = 0.9$). This suggests that the parietal cell density remains relatively constant. The same appears to be true for peptic cells. This makes measurements of parietal cell density an unreliable indicator of parietal cell mass.

Hypophysectomy produced a marked regression in the growth of gastric mucosa which was independent of the effect on somatic growth. The parietal cell population was similarly effected.

There has been much interest in situations that might lead to parietal cell hyperplasia. Partial duodenal stenosis in rats produces an increase in the number of both parietal cells and chief cells (19). In more recent work Crean has found that gastrin pentapeptide administered daily to rats was followed by a pure parietal cell hyperplasia, a possible analogue to work hyperplasia (20). He reported that both duodenal stenosis and gastrin pentapeptide increased acid secretion. Obstruction of gastric pouches in dogs also led to hypersecretion of acid (87).

Since the rat may be something of a maverick in gastric secretion, it is comforting to know that parietal cell populations increase exponentially with growth in beagle dogs (93). There was a 220-fold increase in the total number of parietal cells between birth and maturity. Both surface area and the mucosal thickness increased with age, but there was only a slight increase in parietal cell density.

Properties of Gastric Mucosa

The gastric mucosa exhibits a characteristic potential difference with reference to the serosal surface. In the body of the human stomach, this amounts to -44 millivolts, falling to -35 in the pyloric antrum. In the duodenal bulb the PD was -7 mv, while in the esophagus it fell to 10 to 39 mv (34). Potential measurements have been used as a method for determining the transition from duodenum to stomach (3,7) and stomach to esophagus (70). The area of change in the esophagus correlated better with the presence of parietal cells than with the junction between stratified squamous and columnar epithelium.

The gastric mucosa exhibits striking differences in permeability. Water movements can be interpreted to indicate the existence of two species of pores; 93 per cent had a radius of 2.5 Å, in the range of those found in cell membranes. Seven per cent had a radius of 60 Å, which might occur between cells (31). Villegas postulated two populations of pores in frog gastric mucosa (97). He interpreted his results as indicating that the smaller pores limited bulk flow and were widened by the action of histamine. The large pores, in series with the smaller, limited diffusion, and were unaffected by histamine.

Davenport has carried out an extensive study of the limitations on ion movements in the stomach and the effects of mucosal injury (24). He found that in the normal dog stomach the movement of sodium from blood to lumen and of hydrogen ion from lumen to blood was restricted. However, when the mucosa was injured, hydrogen ion diffused out of the lumen and sodium moved freely into the lumen.

A hoary subject of debate is the question of why the stomach does not digest itself. The late Franklin Hollander proposed that the mucus lying on the surface of the gastric mucosa and the surface epithelial cells themselves functioned as a two-component barrier to the digestive properties of gastric juice. He supported this hypothesis with evidence that the mucosa responded to local application of injurious solutions by first producing more mucus and then, in response to increased dosage of the toxins, shedding surface epithelial cells into the lumen (53).

Methods of Study of Gastric Secretion

Certain technical procedures are used so commonly in the study of gastric secretion that it is necessary to become familiar with them. The determination of hydrogen ion concentration would seem to be a simple task. Unfortunately gastric content is almost always contaminated with other ionic species, organic material, and sometimes even food. Therefore hydrogen ion activity is what is measured with glass electrodes. At pH values near 7 this remains the standard practice. However, under maximal stimulation with histamine, insulin, or gastrin, the gastric pH usually falls to between 0.9 and 1.2. It has been common practice to determine "hydrogen ion concentration" under these circumstances by titration with sodium hydroxide. More biophysically oriented workers have urged that hydrogen ion activity be determined with a glass electrode and corrected to concentration by use of standard tables (74). However, in working at concentrations of HCl of the order of 100 to 160 mEq/L, it is necessary to use specially prepared standard solutions to calibrate the pH meter (76). Actually in this range there is little error introduced by using titratable acidity providing one can determine a proper end point (pH 7 to 7.4), preferably by use of a pH meter rather than an indicator.

Rune (82) introduced a fascinating approach to the determination of acid secretion in response to a meal in man. By arterial puncture he determined the total loss of hydrogen ion from extracellular fluid. After correcting for bicarbonate loss from the pancreas he calculated the total hydrogen ion secreted without the need for intubation. He found that the response correlated well with the maximum response to histamine determined by aspiration.

For many purposes, particularly in assessing the importance of specific variables, it is useful to obtain gastric secretion from fundic mucosa uncontaminated by saliva, duodenal content, or pyloric secretions. For this purpose, portions of the stomach can be isolated from the main stomach (36). Figure 4-5 shows some of the classic preparations. In general, pouches may be of three types: vagally innervated (Pavlov pouch), vagally denervated but with sympathetic fibers still intact (Heidenhain pouch), and denervated or transplanted pouches. Vagal denervation is accomplished by transecting the wall of the stomach. It is preserved by constructing a septum using the mucosa but leaving the remainder of the wall intact. Similar techniques may be applied to antral pouches. The assumption is made that pouches reflect accurately events in the main stomach. However, it is known that many Pavlov pouches have a marked reduction in the number of vagal fibers and the effect of prolonged diversion of gastric content is still unknown.

In vitro methods offer the opportunity to study gastric mucosa as a membrane; they have given many insights into the mechanisms of gastric secretion. In order to ensure adequate oxygenation, a thin membrane is essential. Frog gastric mucosa has served this purpose. Figure 4-6 illustrates a typical preparation. In order to characterize transport one must be able to control the composition of the solutions bathing the two sides of the mucosa, to measure the potential difference across the mucosa, and to measure the current flowing when the mucosal PD is cancelled out by passing a current in the opposite direction. The current that can be recorded under these circumstances (the short-circuit current) reflects the movement of ions against an electrochemical gradient (if the concentrations of the solutions bathing the two surfaces of the membrane is the same).

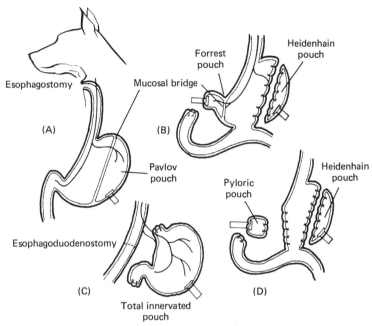

FIGURE 4-5. Illustration of the various types of innervated and denervated fundic and pyloric pouches. (From D. F. Magee. *Gastro-intestinal Physiology.* Springfield, Ill.: Charles C Thomas, Publisher, 1962.)

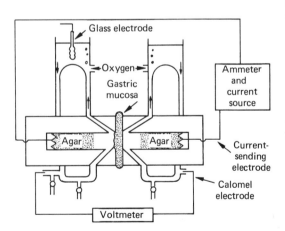

FIGURE 4-6. Apparatus for the study of a gastric mucosal segment in a chamber. Epithelial surface is to the left. (From S. Emås, K. G. Swan, and E. D. Jacobson. Methods of studying gastric secretion. In: *Handbook of Physiology,* Section 6: Alimentary Tract. Vol. 2: Secretion. Edited by C. F. Code. Washington, D.C.: American Physiological Society, 1967, pp. 743–758.)

Composition of Gastric Secretion

ELECTROLYTES

As in the case of the salivary glands, gastric secretion is a composite of the products of several cell types, each subjected to variable controlling factors. The problem is further compounded in the stomach by the mixture of secretions from three surfaces—the fundic glands, the pyloric glands, and the surface epithelium. In the normal human, swallowed saliva and regurgitated duodenal content further modify gastric content. Direct measurement of parietal cell secretion has not been possible. Various attempts have been made at determining the composition of the nonparietal secretions. Acid-free content from Heidenhain pouches in dogs (15), secretion from flaps of fundic mucosa in anesthetized dogs after the intraarterial injection of acetylcholine (2), and secretion from explants of gastric mucosa in rats containing only surface epithelial cells (98) have been analyzed and shown to approximate the composition of extracellular fluid. Similarly, secretion from pyloric pouches in dogs approaches the electrolyte composition of plasma (44). The main variable has been the bicarbonate concentration, which is frequently less than that of plasma.

Since Pavlov, the most popular concept to explain the variable composition of gastric secretion has been the two-component hypothesis (55). This theory postulates a secretion of hydrogen ion at a concentration of about 170 mEq/L (primary acidity). The amount of hydrogen secreted is a function of the number of parietal cells secreting, since it is usually assumed that parietal cells secrete in an all-or-none fashion. Acid is then diluted by the nonparietal secretions. The latter are often assumed to secrete at a steady rate, so that the variable is the number of parietal cells secreting at any one time. Makhlouf is probably the most vehement champion of this point of view at present (66). Performing innumerable studies on himself and McManus he has constructed elegant mathematical models which are compatible with such a hypothesis.

However, it would be surprising in the face of such an extreme concentration gradient if some hydrogen ion did not re-enter the mucosa. Teorell placed this on a quantitative basis by trapping hydrogen ions with a glycine buffer (42). With this technique he obtained values for primary acidity far exceeding 170 mEq/L. Overhalt and Pollard obtained greater acid outputs in man with a glycine buffer (79). Rosenmann postulated that the parietal cells separated off NaCl from the plasma and converted a variable portion to HCl (55). Finally, Hirschowitz, influenced by renal physiologists, suggested that the chief cells in the depths of the fundic glands secreted sodium chloride and pepsin (55). This solution passed through the gland and at the level of the parietal cells exchanged hydrogen ion for sodium. Individual experiments can be cited supporting each of the foregoing theories, but none can account satisfactorily for all observations. Hunt (53) has called for a quantitative formulation of a combined Teorell-Hollander (two-component) hypothesis (55).

The material presented already should give some indication of the difficulty in obtaining good collections of gastric content in man. Once obtained, such data can be used for theoretical considerations. The hardy survival of Ihre's results, obtained in 1938, and the seemingly endless permutations of Makhlouf and McManus are good examples of this kind of research (56,69). Fisher and Hunt used Ihre's data to show a variation in the composition of the nonparietal component of secretion obtained after stimulation with insulin compared to that after histamine (38).

One observation stands out from the human studies; there is less variability obtained with maximal stimulation than under basal or resting or interdigestive conditions. In man, interdigestive secretion of hydrogen ion commonly ranges up to 2 mEq/hour. Collections over the 12 hours from 8:00 p.m. to 8:00 a.m. vary around 600 ml and a concentration of 39 mEq/L. There are significant differences related to age and sex. Coefficients of variation often reach 25 per cent. On the other hand, maximal stimulation with histamine, histalog (betazole), gastrin, gastrin pentapeptide, and gastrin tetrapeptide all result in a similar value for acid secretory capacity correlated with the parietal cell mass (65). Results are reproducible in the same individual within 10 per cent. It should be noted that after a year of repeated gastric intubations, one of the two famous Edinburgh subjects ceased to secrete acid in the basal state and continued to be achlorhydric in the absence of stimulation for the subsequent 8 months. This suggests that parietal cell population is not spontaneously active but reacts only to stimulation (68).

Several investigators have pointed out the advantages of determining maximal acid output with continuous intravenous infusions of histamine, and Moore has offered a scheme for calculating maximal secretion from several points on a dose-response curve (75).

It is of interest to compare the maximal secretory capacity of the stomach to that of the pancreas. Using submaximal stimulation with secretin in man, Janowitz and his colleagues found that the pancreas produced sufficient bicarbonate to neutralize the maximally stimulated acid response to histamine (8).

Other ionic constituents in gastric secretion include chloride and potassium. Chloride is usually present in concentrations greater than hydrogen ion—the so-called neutral chloride. According to Rosenmann's theory, the chloride concentration should remain constant over a range of hydrogen ion concentrations, and it sometimes does (55). Potassium concentrations in gastric juice, like those in saliva, rise transiently with various stimuli, but thereafter show a parallelism with hydrogen ion which suggests that a portion of the potassium emerges from the parietal cell in parallel with HCl. It should be noted that the concentration exceeds that in plasma.

MACROMOLECULES

Gastric secretion contains at least two proteases—pepsin, with a molecular weight of 42,500 and a pH optimum of 2.0, and gastricsin, with a molecular weight of 31,000 and a pH optimum of 3.2. Some differences in amino acid sequence have been demonstrated between the two molecules, as well as differences in their action on substrates. It remains to be settled whether they arise from different pepsinogens within the gastric mucosa or share a common precursor (94).

Piper et al. (81) found eight nonproteolytic enzymes in human gastric content, collected after neutralizing the gastric juice by intragastric instillation of sodium carbonate. All were known to be intracellular enzymes, including transaminases, phosphatases, and glucuronidase. It is not known how they enter the stomach—by secretion, by shedding of cells, or by leaking out of the cells. They were always present in higher concentrations in the gastric mucosa than in gastric content.

Gastric secretion contains lipolytic activity. According to Davenport, there is a tributyrinase (23). Recently, activity against trioctanoin has been found with a significant degree of hydrolysis occurring in the human stomach (17).

Intrinsic factor, necessary for the absorption of vitamin B_{12}, is present in gastric secretion. Active material separated from human gastric juice had a molecular weight of 100,000, but the biologic activity is retained by much smaller molecules (59).

Like other digestive secretions, gastric juice contains an inhibitor, in this case directed against acid secretion. Gastrone has been shown to consist of at least two materials—a mucuslike substance with a molecular weight of over 100,000 and containing much carbohydrate, and a nondialyzable glyco-polypeptide or glycoprotein with a molecular weight between 10,000 and 40,000. The first has weak inhibitory properties and is resistant to peptic digestion so that it may function in acid gastric juice. The second is a more potent inhibitor and has some of the properties of globulin. It is degraded by proteolytic enzymes and is probably responsible for the inhibitory properties of anacid gastric juice (37).

Finally, gastric secretion contains that conspicuous but difficult to analyze substance mucus (54). "Visible" mucus is a water-insoluble complex of glyco-proteins, serum proteins, and pepsinogen or pepsin. "Dissolved" mucus is composed of similar materials. The relationship between the two is unknown. Proteins and the protein portion of glycoproteins constitute 60 to 80 per cent of the nondialyzable substance of gastrointestinal secretions. The principal mucosubstances in gastric secretions and gastric mucosa are glycoproteins. Workers in the field rely upon measurements of amino sugars, hexoses, and sialic acid to quantitate their results. Glass comments, "with few exceptions, none of the above techniques have provided a degree of resolution and purification acceptable to the current requirements of modern chemistry" (43).

Perhaps the best-known biologically active components of gastric mucus are the blood group substances. No conclusions can be drawn as yet about the influence of blood group status on the composition of secretion (54).

The acid mucopolysaccharides constitute a smaller fraction of hog gastric mucosal scrapings than the blood group active glycoproteins. The only pure AMPS which have been isolated from mucosal scrapings are heparin and chondroitin sulfate.

Mechanism of Formation of Gastric Secretion

HYDROCHLORIC ACID

The formation of hydrochloric acid can be viewed from several levels (25). Considering the changes in blood passing through the stomach in vivo, gastric venous blood is lower in chloride concentration and higher in bicarbonate than arterial blood. Using isolated frog gastric mucosa, Davies found that acid secretion on the mucosal side was coupled with an equivalent release of bicarbonate on the serosal side (26,27). Removal of CO_2 from the serosal solution with acid-secreting mucosae resulted in perforating ulcers, presumably from failure to convert hydroxyl ions to bicarbonate.

As noted previously spontaneous acid secretion probably does not occur in man, yet it is interesting that some frog gastric mucosae will secrete in vitro only during certain seasons of the year. Most investigators of the mechanism of HCl secretion have turned to in vitro preparations to study this problem.

As with other transport processes, the secretion of HCl must be viewed in relation to the electrochemical gradients present in the gastric mucosa. The electronegativity of the mucosa with respect to the serosa is a property of the mucosa itself. It is related to the active transport of chloride ion. Most workers favor the concept of two separate electrogenic "pumps"—one for hydrogen ion and the other for chloride. In frog gastric mucosa, Villegas found a membrane potential of -49.2 mv in the surface epithelial cells which varied in response to the concentration of potassium in the mucosa. The membrane potential of the parietal cells was -17.7 mv. Replacing chloride with sulfate abolished the asymmetry of potentials across the parietal cells (96).

Studies on movement of individual ions across the gastric mucosa show that chloride moves by active transport (52), passive diffusion, and exchange diffusion (32) across the mucosal surface. Water moves in response to diffusion and to a limited degree in response to osmotic gradients. Hydrostatic pressure of capillary blood causes some water flow. This can be demonstrated in the mucosal flap preparation, mounted in a chamber, by applying a force equal to the hydrostatic pressure to the mucosal surface (2,72).

The transport of hydrogen ions by the parietal cells is a very specific mechanism, and no other cation can be substituted in its place. In contrast, a variety of anions may substitute for chloride. The mechanism by which potassium ions enter gastric secretion is unknown (27).

In vitro preparations also permit study of the importance of solutions bathing the serosal or nutrient side of the mucosa. Sodium is essential for frog mucosa to maintain a potential difference and to secrete acid (34). There is an active transport system in nonsecreting cat gastric mucosa for moving sodium and chloride independently (61). Removal of calcium from the nutrient secretion of frog gastric mucosa reduces acid secretion. This may be related to a coincident widening of intercellular spaces (85).

The cellular metabolism concerned with acid secretion is under intensive study. A variety of enzymes have been identified by histochemical or chemical techniques in gastric mucosa. One of the first was carbonic anhydrase. Davies suggested that it was the function of this enzyme to catalyze the hydration of carbon dioxide and thereby protect the gastric mucosa from the action of hydroxyl ions released in the formation of hydrogen ion from water (26). In humans, parenteral administration of the carbonic anhydrase inhibitor acetazolamide will inhibit acid secretion (58). Sulfhydryl inhibitors also inhibit acid secretion. The activity of a series of cellular enzymes of rat parietal cells was determined by histochemical techniques and repeated after exposure to sulfhydryl inhibitors. There was a significant reduction in activity (91).

Succinic oxidase is another enzyme system present in high concentrations in parietal cells and possibly concerned with acid secretion. Perhaps the enzyme of greatest interest is an ATPase associated with the tubular membranes of gastric mucosal cell microsomes (28). Its activity is inhibited by thiocyanate, which also inhibits acid secretion, but it is not stimulated by sodium and potassium as are many other ATPases. Durbin and Kasbekar (33) suggest that the enzyme may be concerned with the translocation of chloride and bicarbonate.

The substrates for release of the energy required by acid secretion include carbohydrates in the isolated mouse stomach (22) and the water-soluble salts of short- and medium-chain fatty acids and ketones in the frog (1). Amino acids and the intermediates of the tricarboxylic acid cycle were without effect.

The formation of hydrochloric acid in mammals requires oxygen. The ratio of hydrogen ion secreted to mol of oxygen consumed is a measure of efficiency and may suggest the characteristics of the metabolic process. Unfortunately parietal cells are only one component of gastric mucosa, and the extent to which other cells participate in oxygen consumption is unknown. ATP is a likely candidate for an energy source in acid secretion. Forte calculated that 1.5 equivalents of hydrogen ion could be secreted for each mol of ATP utilized. In general a simple redox pump would not satisfy the characteristics of the system (39).

MECHANISM FOR THE SECRETION OF PEPSIN

The mechanism by which digestive enzymes are secreted by cells has been discussed in the case of salivary amylase. The differences between the serous cells and chief cells lie in the fact that the digestive enzyme is present within the secretory granule in an inactive precursor form—a true zymogen. Figure 4-7 illustrates Hirschowitz' concept of pepsinogen secretion (50). The zymogen granules represent a storage form, and secretion of pepsinogen can occur in their absence. He suggests that the initial increase in output of pepsin in response to a variety of stimuli is the result of an asymmetry of cellular response in time rather than a simple washout in acid secretion of preformed enzyme. As with other proteins, synthesis must be distinguished from extrusion. Villarreal found no evidence for synthesis of pepsinogen in isolated frog gastric mucosa in the presence of amino acids in the bath, even though pepsin was secreted in response to stimulation (95).

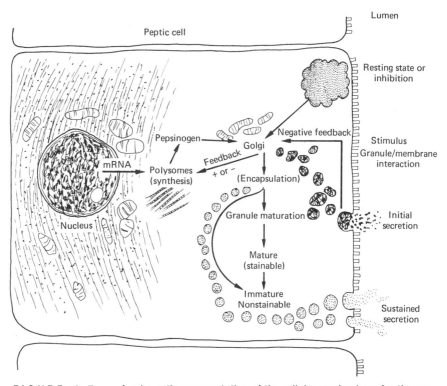

FIGURE 4-7. A schematic representation of the cellular mechanisms for the synthesis, storage, and secretion of pepsinogen. (From B. I. Hirschowitz. Secretion of pepsinogen. In: *Handbook of Physiology*, Section 6: Alimentary Tract. Vol. 2: Secretion. Edited by C. F. Code. Washington, D.C.: American Physiological Society, 1967, pp. 889–918.)

There is an interesting exocrine-endocrine partition of pepsinogen result-ing in the presence of a level of pepsinogen in the blood. The latter in turn leads to excretion of peptic activity in the urine—uropepsin.

MECHANISM OF MUCOUS SECRETION

Very little is known of the mechanism of mucous secretion. Electron microscopists describe three morphologic mechanisms: fusion of the mucous granule with the apical cell membrane, solubilization of the mucus and passage through an intact membrane, and extrusion of the entire cell together with its mucous granules (57). The biochemistry of this process is unknown. By analogy with the formation of blood glycoproteins in the liver, microsomes are the site of synthesis (54).

Control of Gastric Secretion

CELLULAR CONTROL OF HYDROCHLORIC ACID SECRETION

Harris and Alonso (46) found that cyclic AMP stimulated acid secretion by frog gastric mucosa in vitro, so this ubiquitous excitant may play a role in gastric acid secretion. Bannister reported that oligomycin had little effect on frog acid secretion but reduced oxygen consumption, while dinitrophenol reduced acid secretion but stimulated oxygen consumption, suggesting that the synthesis of ATP was not necessary for the separation of hydrogen and hydroxyl ions from water (9).

The prime candidates for the excitant of acid secretion at the cellular level are acteylcholine, gastrin, and histamine. At present no choice can be made for man. The evidence for histamine comes largely from studies in rats which may be unique (16).

CELLULAR CONTROL OF PEPSIN SECRETION

Hirschowitz suggests that pepsinogen synthesis is under control of a negative feedback system so that when secretion is inhibited, synthesis is slowed as well (50). The presence of an increased amount of zymogen granules in the cell would presumably act as a signal. Similarly depletion of zymogen granules would stimulate synthesis—positive feedback. However, synthesis can apparently accelerate and equal secretory rates over periods of stimulation. The evidence for these systems is fragmentary. Atropine inhibits secretion without effect on synthesis (48).

In contrast to acid secretion, acetylcholine is the leading candidate for a cellular excitant, but the species differences in response to gastrin and histamine are even greater. Hyperventilation in man produces stimulation of pepsin secretion independently of the vagus nerves and presumably acts directly on the chief cells (50).

GASTRIC CONTROL OF GASTRIC SECRETION OF HYDROCHLORIC ACID

The stomach has three main mechanisms for controlling acid secretion—the autonomic nervous system, hormones, and the circulation. It is evident that there is joint involvement under many circumstances. In the body of the stomach, the only local system of control is that of local nervous reflexes. Distention can elicit an acid secretory response presumably through cholinergic nerves.

The pyloric antrum contains a more complex system. Receptors responding to distention exist in the antrum. Elwin and Urnas found that alcohol, amino acids, and dipeptides acted on chemoreceptors in the antrum (35). This observation may explain the excitatory effects of food in the stomach. The afferent pathway involves an intermediate ganglion. The efferent path centers on the cells producing the hormone gastrin. After sixty years, Gregory and his associates purified and later synthesized gastrin (41). It is a polypeptide containing seventeen amino acids, of which the C-terminal tetrapeptide is essential for its physiologic action. Figure 4-8 shows the structure of gastrin in man. Acetylcholine applied to the antral mucosa stimulates gastrin release by acting directly on the gastrin-producing cell. On the other hand, acids in the antrum lowering the pH to less than 3 act directly upon the gastrin-producing cell to inhibit release without the intervention of a neural pathway. Figure 4-9 illustrates the schema (84).

On this purely gastric regulatory mechanism, the parasympathetic division of the autonomic nervous system, through the vagi, impose another level of control. As already mentioned, afferent fibers in the vagus respond to changes in osmotic pressure, pH, and mechanical tension. Efferent fibers in the vagi synapse with ganglion cells in the submucosal plexus and by means of the local nervous control system already presented excite parietal cells directly

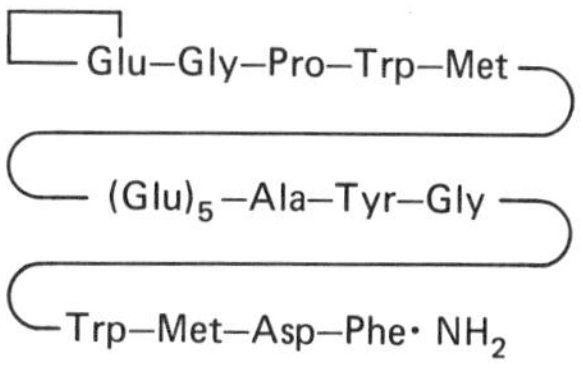

Glu–Gly–Pro–Trp–Met

$(Glu)_5$–Ala–Tyr–Gly

Trp–Met–Asp–Phe· NH_2

M. W. = 2114

FIGURE 4-8.

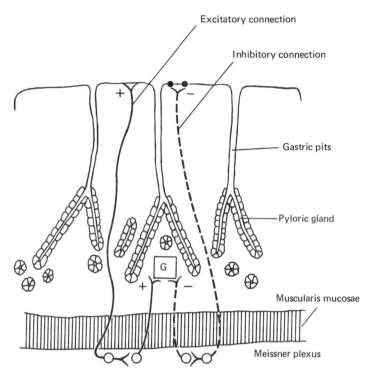

FIGURE 4-9.   Diagram to show postulated nervous pathways in the antral mucosa. A synapse has been shown in the excitatory pathway, since investigations with hexamethonium support the possibility that this exists. (From M. Redford and B. Schofield. *J. Physiol. London* **180**: 304–320, 1965.)

or through the release of gastrin (*40*). Figure 4-10 shows this system in diagram.

Under most circumstances, excitation of gastric secretion is associated with an increase in mucosal blood flow even though total gastric blood flow remains unchanged (*73,92*). There remains the possibility that adrenergic neuro-humoral transmitters such as norepinephrine may exert at least some inhibitory action on secretion indirectly through limiting mucosal blood flow (*88*).

EXTRAGASTRIC CONTROL OF GASTRIC SECRETION OF HYDROCHLORIC ACID

The main sources of control outside the stomach are the small intestine, the central nervous system, and the endocrine glands. Distention of the small intestine may lead to excitation or inhibition of acid secretion. Excitation seems to be dependent upon hormonal mechanisms of an unknown nature—"intestinal gastrin." Acid in the duodenum inhibits acid secretion. This, too, seems to be humorally mediated, although intact nerves may increase the sensitivity

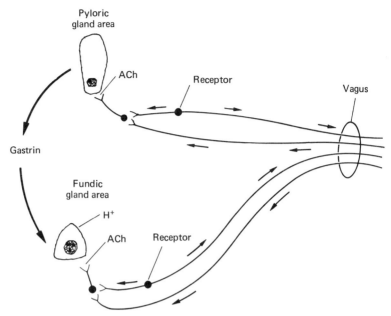

FIGURE 4-10. Diagrammatic representation of the intramural and vagal inner-uation of gastric mucosa. (From M. I. Grossman. *Physiologist* **6:** 349, 1963.)

of the mechanism. In the dog, the acid receptors appear to be confined to the duodenal bulb (5). It is interesting in man that only the bulb contains fluid with a fluctuating pH, reaching levels of less than 2 after meals or stimulation of acid secretion. (3,7).

In the dog, secretin, a polypeptide containing 27 amino acid residues, and present in the intestinal mucosa, can account for most of the antisecretory effects of acid in the duodenum. Secretin is also effective in this regard in man (4). Cross-circulation experiments in man during acidification of the duodenum also suggest that a humoral agent is released under the circumstances which inhibits acid secretion (60).

Fat in the intestine also inhibits acid secretion. This is the basis for the hypothetical inhibitory hormone enterogastrone. In dogs, fat is effective in the jejunum in releasing an inhibitory mechanism in contrast to acid. The mechanism of action of fat remains uncertain (6).

The central nervous control of acid secretion seems clear from evidence in behavioral studies and neurophysiologic experiments (12). The device of sham feeding (swallowing food which escapes through an esophagostomy) can elicit an acid secretory response equal to that of maximal histamine stimulation. It is abolished by vagotomy or removal of the gastrin-secreting mucosa (78). This indicates that the initial stimulation of acid secretion upon the ingestion of food depends upon vagal release of gastrin.

Insulin hypoglycemia or cellular glucopenia induced with 2-deoxy-D-glucose stimulates neurons extending from the hypothalamus to the vagal nuclei with a resultant excitation of acid secretion. The excitation is blocked by vagotomy or prevention of the glucopenia (49).

In the rat the same areas of the hypothalamus concerned with the control of food intake also influence gastric secretion in an appropriate fashion— lesions or stimulation resulting in increased food intake increase acid secretion, while those producing inhibition of food intake decrease interdigestive secretion. Higher levels of the visceral nervous system in primates seem to be involved in the inhibition of acid secretion that occurs in response to acute stressful stimuli, possibly through the release of vasoconstrictive catechol amines (89,90). Prolonged stressful situations may lead to loss of normal diurnal cycles of acid secretion with a net increase in 24-hour acid output (12).

The endocrine glands as a whole seem to exert little control over gastric secretion under normal circumstances. The effect of hypophysectomy on gastric secretion has already been mentioned, and adrenalectomy in man is similarly associated with a diminished secretory capacity (18). These may be considered as examples of the permissive role of the endocrines. Pancreatectomy may be followed by hypersecretion of acid in dogs but this seems to result from lack of the digestive function of pancreatic enzymes rather than a hormonal factor (14). Hypercalcemia, both in hyperparathyroidism and after calcium infusions, seems to induce an increase in basal secretion in man, dependent upon cholinergic pathways (10, 11, 77).

CONTROL OF PEPSIN SECRETION

In general pepsin secretion and acid secretion run parallel in man (67,83). This follows from the increases in volume of gastric juice rather than changes in concentration of pepsin. The outputs of pepsin after histamine and gastrin in man suggest that peptic and parietal cell masses are present in the same ratios in different human subjects.

Striking dissociation in acid-pepsin secretion has been reported after acetazolamide, cholecystokinin, and secretin in dogs (47). Acid secretion was inhibited and pepsin secretion stimulated. The significance of these observations for man remains to be seen.

CONTROL OF INTRINSIC FACTOR SECRETION

Intrinsic factor activity in the gastric juice of man is stimulated by histamine, but in comparison to acid output, it rises to an early peak and then falls despite sustained acid output. An anticholinergic agent had no significant effect on the output of intrinsic factor under these circumstances (30,99).

CONTROL OF MUCOUS SECRETION

According to Menguy, mucous secretion from antral pouches in dogs is unchanged after meals, increased by serotonin and acidification of the antrum, and decreased by vagal or cholinergic stimuli and corticotropin (29,71). Changes in the composition of mucus occurred after antral acidification.

SUMMARY OF THE CONTROL OF ACID SECRETION

The local control of acid secretion functions as an autoregulatory system in the absence of overriding external factors. Gastrin release excites the fundic glands to secrete acid, but a low antral pH leads to cessation of gastrin release. Intestinal control factors are largely inhibitory. This is also true of the central nervous system, with the striking exception of areas concerned also with the increase in food intake. An important but unexplored area is the role of the vasomotor system in the control of acid secretion, particularly through vaso-constrictor mechanisms.

Function of the Stomach in Man

The only vital component of gastric secretion in man is intrinsic factor. In its absence vitamin B_{12} absorption fails and normal hematopoeisis cannot occur. Inability of the stomach to secrete acid or pepsin per se does not seem to influence general body function.

Pathophysiology

Much of the symptomatology of peptic ulcer disease and almost all of its therapy is based upon physiologic considerations. The subject is covered at length elsewhere (see monograph edited by Skoryna). It is sufficient to note that secretion may be reduced by anticholinergic drugs or by cutting the vagi or removing the gastrin-forming areas or acid-secreting glands. So far, attempts to implicate defective protective mechanisms such as mucus or the inhibitory intestinal mechanism have failed. Perhaps the most elegant success of patho-physiology is the discovery of a nonbeta-islet-cell tumor that produces a polypeptide similar if not identical with gastrin. These patients manifest massive hypersecretion and severe peptic ulcer disease.

Summary of Physiology of Gastric Secretion

The gastric mucosa has a maximum secretory capacity of about 10 mEq/hr per 500 million parietal cells. In the absence of stimulation the output in man is near zero. The energy for HCl secretion comes primarily from oxidative metabolism and may involve adenosine triphosphate. Enzymes such as carbonic anhydrase, succinic oxidase, and an ATPase are probably involved, but the specific pathway is unknown. Excitants of gastric secretion act on mechanoreceptors and chemoreceptors within the gastrointestinal tract and upon receptors within the nervous system. As a result, the hormone gastrin may be released from the pyloric antrum, or impulses traveling over the vagus nerves may reach the parietal cells directly. The release of gastrin is inhibited by acid in the antrum, so that excitation via gastrin release leads to inhibition of release. Acid in the duodenum releases a humoral agent, possibly secretin, which inhibits gastrin-stimulated secretion. In general, pepsin secretion follows acid secretion, but humoral agents that inhibit acid secretion may stimulate pepsin secretion. Intrinsic factor follows acid secretion to a degree and shares the same cell of origin in man. Mucus remains a great enigma, from the point of view of both its chemistry and its physiologic control. Blood flow to the mucosa usually increases when acid output increases.

References

1. Alonso, D., K. Nigon, I. Door, and J. B. Harris. Energy sources for gastric secretion: substrates. *Am. J. Physiol.* **212:** 992–1000, 1967.
2. Altamirano, M. Alkaline secretion produced by intra-arterial acetycholine. *J. Physiol. London* **168:** 787–803, 1963.
3. Andersson, S., and M. I. Grossman. Profile of pH, pressure and potential difference as gastroduodenal junction in man. *Gastroenterology* **49:** 364–371, 1965.
4. Andersson, S., and M. I. Grossman. Effects of histalog and secretin on gastroduodenal profile of pH, potential difference and pressure in man. *Gastroenterology* **51:** 10–17, 1966.
5. Andersson, S., G. Nilsson, and B. Uvnas. Effect of acid in proximal and distal duodenal pouches on gastric secretory responses to gastrin and histamine. *Acta Physiol. Scand.* **71:** 368–378, 1967.
6. Andersson, S. Gastric and duodenal mechanisms inhibiting gastric secretion of acid. In: *Handbook of Physiology.* Section 6: Alimentary Tract. Vol. II: Secretion. Edited by C. F. Code. Washington D.C.: American Physiological Society, 1967, pp. 865–878.
7. Archambault, A. P., R. A. Rovelstad, and H. C. Carlson. In situ pH of duodenal bulb contents in normal and duodenal ulcer subjects. *Gastroenterology* **52:** 940–947, 1967.
8. Banks, P. A., W. P. Dyck, D. A. Dreiling, and H. D. Janowitz. Secretory capacity of stomach and pancreas in man. *Gastroenterology* **53:** 575–578, 1967.
9. Bannister, W. H. The effect of oligomycin and some nitrophenols on acid secretion and oxygen uptake by gastric mucosa of the frog. *J. Physiol. London* **186:** 89–96, 1966.
10. Barreras, R. F., and R. M. Donaldson, Jr. Gastric secretion during hypercalcemia in man. *Gastroenterology* **50:** 881, 1966.

11. Barreras, R. F., and R. M. Donaldson, Jr. Effects of induced hypercalcemia on human gastric secretion. *Gastroenterology* **52:** 670–675, 1967.

11b Bralow, S. P., and S. A. Komarov. Parietal cell mass and distribution in stomachs of Wistar rats. *Am. J. Physiol.* **203:** 550–552, 1962.

12. Brooks, F. P. Central neural control of acid secretion. In: *Handbook of Physiology.* Section 6: Alimentary Tract. Vol. II: Secretion. Edited by C. F. Code. Washington, D.C.: American Physiological Society, 1967, pp. 805–826.

13. Card, W. I., and I. N. Marks. The relationship between the acid output of the stomach following "maximal" histamine stimulation and the parietal cell mass. *Clin. Sci.* **19:** 147–163, 1960

14. Chey, C. Y., and S. H. Lorber. Influence of pancreas on gastric secretion in dogs. *Am. J. Physiol.* **212:** 252–260, 1967.

15. Clarke, S. D., D. W. Neill, and R. B. Welbourn. The effects of corticotrophin and corticoids on secretion from denervated gastric pouches in dogs. *Gut* **I:** 36–43, 1960.

16. Code, C. F. Histamine and gastric secretion: a later look 1955–1965. *Fed. Proc.* **24:** 1311–1321, 1965.

17. Cohen, M., R. G. H. Morgan, and A. F. Hofmann. The lipolytic activity of human gastric juice. *Fed. Proc.* **27:** 574, 1968.

18. Cooke, A. R. Role of adrenocortical steroids in the regulation of gastric secretion. *Gastroenterology* **52:** 272–281, 1967.

19. Crean, G. P. Observations on the regulation of the growth of the gastric mucosa. In: *Gastric Secretion. Mechanisms and Control,* edited by T. K. Shnitka, J. A. L. Gilbert, and R. C. Harrison. New York: Pergamon Press. 1967, pp. 33–43.

20. Crean, G. P., R. D. E. Rumsey, D. F. Hogg, and M. W. Marshall. Experimental hyperplasia of the gastric mucosa. In: *The Physiology of Gastric Secretion.* Edited by L. S. Semb and J. Myren. Baltimore: Williams and Wilkins Co., 1968, pp. 82–85.

21. Croft, D. N., D. J. Pollock, and N. F. Coghill. Cell loss from human gastric mucosa measured by the estimation of deoxyribonucleic acid (DNA) in gastric washings. *Gut* **7:** 333–343, 1966.

22. Davenport, H. W. Metabolic aspects of gastric acid secretion. In: *Metabolic Aspects of Transport Across Cell Membranes.* Edited by Q. R. Murphy. Madison: University of Wisconsin Press, 1957, pp. 295–302.

23. Davenport, H. W. *The Physiology of the Digestive Tract* (2nd ed.). Chicago: Year Book Medical Publishers, 1966, pp. 96–97.

24. Davenport, H. W. Physiological structure of the gastric mucosa. In: *Handbook of Physiology.* Section 6: Alimentary Tract. Vol. 11: Secretion. Edited by C. F. Code. Washington, D.C.: American Physiological Society, 1967, pp. 759–779.

25. Davson, H. *A Textbook of General Physiology* (3rd ed.). Boston: Little Brown & Co., 1964, pp. 539–558.

26. Davies, R. E. Gastric hydrochloric acid production—The present position. In: *Metabolic Aspects of Transport Across Cell Membranes.* Edited by Q. R. Murphy. Madison: University of Wisconsin Press, 1957, pp. 277–293.

27. Davies, R. E., and J. Forte. Secretion of acid by the stomach. In: *Pathophysiology of Peptic Ulcer.* Edited by S. C. Skoryna. Philadelphia: J. B. Lippincott Co., 1963, pp. 3–22.

28. Davies, R. E. The metabolism of gastric mucosa during the secretion of hydro-

chloric acid. In: *Gastric Secretion: Mechanisms and Control.* Edited by T. K. Shnitka, J. A. L. Gilbert, and R. C. Harrison. New York: Pergamon Press, 1967, pp. 45–51.

29. Desbaillets, L., and R. Menguy. Inhibition of gastric mucous secretion by ACTH: An experimental study. *Am. J. Dig. Dis.* **12:** 582–588, 1967.

30. Dotevall, G., A. Walan, and A. Weinfeld. Effect of 1-hyoxcyamine on gastric secretion of acid and intrinsic factor in man. *Gut* **8:** 276–280, 1967.

31. Durbin, R. P., H. Frank, and A. K. Solomon. Water flow through frog gastric mucosa. *J. Gen. Physiol.* **39:** 535–551, 1956.

32. Durbin, R. P., S. Kitahara, K. Stahlmann, and E. Heinz. Exchange diffusion of chloride in frog gastric mucosa. *Am. J. Physiol.* **207:** 1177–1180, 1964.

33. Durbin, R. P., and D. K. Kasbekar. Adenosine triphosphate and active transport by the stomach. *Fed. Proc.* **24:** 1377–1381, 1965.

34. Durbin, R. P. Electrical potential difference of the gastric mucosa. In: *Handbook of Physiology.* Section 6: Alimentary Tract. Vol. II: Secretion. Edited by C. F. Code. Washington, D.C.: American Physiological Society, 1967, pp. 879–888.

35. Elwin, C. E., and B. Uvnas, Distribution and local release of gastrin. In: *Gastrin.* Edited by M. I. Grossman. Berkeley and Los Angeles: University of California Press, 1967, pp. 69–82.

36. Emas, S., K. G. Swan, and E. D. Jacobson. Methods of studying gastric secretion. In: *Handbook of Physiology.* Section 6: Alimentary Tract. Vol. II: Secretion. Edited by C. F. Code. Washington D.C.: American Physiological Society, 1967, pp. 743–758.

37. Fiasse, R., C. F. Code, and G. B. J. Glass. Fractionation and partial purification of gastrone. *Gastroenterology* **54:** 1018–1031, 1968.

38. Fisher, R. B., and J. N. Hunt. The inorganic components of gastric secretion. *J. Physiol. London* **111:** 138–149, 1950.

39. Forte, J. G. Metabolism of gastric mucosa. *Fed. Proc.* **24:** 1382–1386, 1965.

40. Fyro, B. Reduction of antral and duodenal gastrin activity by electrical vagal stimulation. *Acta Physiol. Scand.* **71:** 334–340, 1967.

41. *Gastroenterology*, Silver Anniversary Issue, edited by T. P. Almy and M. S. Sleisenger. The antrum, gastrin and peptic ulcer. *Gastroenterology* **54:** 723–728, 1968.

42. *Gastroenterology*, Silver Anniversary Issue, edited by T. P. Almy and M. S. Sleisenger. The mechanisms of acid secretion. *Gastroenterology* **54:** 701–714, 1968.

43. Glass, G. B. J. Fractionation of gastric macromolecular materials by electrophoresis, column chromatography and gel filtration: correlative study. In: *Gastric Secretion: Mechanisms and Control.* Edited by T. K. Shnitka, J. A. L. Gilbert, and R. C. Harrison. New York: Pergamon Press, 1967, pp. 187–212.

44. Grossman, M. I. The secretion of the pyloric glands of the dog. XXI Intern. Congr. Physiol. Sci., Buenos Aires. Symp. & Special Lectures, 1959, pp. 226–228.

45. Grossman, M. I. Neural and hormonal stimulation of gastric secretion of acid. In: *Handbook of Physiology.* Section 6: Alimentary Tract. Vol. II: Secretion. Edited by C. F. Code. Washington D.C.: American Physiological Society, 1967, pp. 835–863.

46. Harris, J. B., and D. Alonso. Stimulation of the gastric mucosa by adenosine-3,5-monophosphate. *Fed. Proc.* **24:** 1368–1376, 1965.

47. Heitmann, P., A. M. Jungreis, and H. D. Janowitz. Effect of acetazolamide and cholecystokinin on the secretion of pepsin from histamine-stimulated Heidenhain pouches. *Gastroenterology* **52:** 211–215, 1967.

48. Hirschowitz, B. I., D. K. O'Leary, and I. N. Marks. Effect of atropine on synthesis and secretion of pepsinogen in the rat. *Am. J. Physiol.* **198:** 108–112, 1960.

49. Hirschowitz, B. I., and G. Sachs. Vagal gastric secretory stimulation by 2-deoxy-D-glucose. *Am. J. Physiol.* **209:** 452–460, 1965.

50. Hirschowitz, B. I. Secretion of pepsinogen. In: *Handbook of Physiology.* Section 6: Alimentary Tract. Vol. II: Secretion. Edited by C. F. Code. Washington, D.C.: American Physiological Society, 1967, pp. 889–918.

51. Hoedemaeker, P. J., J. Abels, J. J. Wachters, A. Arends, and H. O. Nieweg. Further investigations about the site of production of Castle's gastric intrinsic factor. *Lab. Invest.* **15:** 1163–1173, 1966.

52. Hogben, C. A. M. Active transport of chloride by isolated frog gastric epithelium. Origin of the gastric mucosal potential. *Am. J. Physiol.* **180:** 641–649, 1955.

53. Hollander, F. The two-component mucosa barrier: Its activity in protecting against peptic ulceration. *Arch. Intern. Med.* **93:** 107–129, 1954.

54. Horowitz, M. I. Mucopolysaccharides and glycoproteins of the alimentary tract. In: *Handbook of Physiology.* Section 6: Alimentary Tract. Vol. II: Secretion. Edited by C. F. Code. Washington D.C.: American Physiological Society, 1967, pp. 1063–1085.

55. Hunt, J. N., and B. Wan. Electrolytes of mammalian gastric juice. In: *Handbook of Physiology.* Section 6: Alimentary Tract. Vol. II: Secretion. Edited by C. F. Code. Washington, D.C.: American Physiological Society, 1967, pp. 781–804.

56. Ihre, B. Human gastric secretion. *Acta Med. Scand.* Suppl. 95, pp. 1–226, 1938.

57. Ito, S. Anatomic structure of the gastric mucosa. In: *Handbook of Physiology.* Section 6: Alimentary Tract. Vol. II: Secretion. Edited by C. F. Code. Washington, D.C.: American Physiological Society, 1967, pp. 705–741.

58. Janowitz, H. D., D. A. Dreiling, and F. Hollander. Inhibition of HCl formation in the human stomach by diamox: The role of carbonic anhydrase in gastric secretion. *J. Clin. Invest.* **34:** 918, 1955.

59. Jeffries, G. H. Gastric secretion of intrinsic factor. In: *Handbook of Physiology.* Section 6: Alimentary Tract Vol. II: Secretion. Edited by C. F. Code. Washington, D.C.: American Physiological Society, 1967, pp. 919–924.

60. Johnston, D., and H. L. Duthie. Inhibition of histamine-stimulated gastric secretion by acid in the duodenum in man. *Gut* **7:** 58–68, 1966.

61. Kitahara, S. Active transport of Na^+ and Cl^- by in vitro non-secreting cat gastric mucosa. *Am. J. Physiol.* **213:** 819–823, 1967.

62. Lipkin, M., P. Sherlock, and B. Bell. Cell proliferation kinetics in the gastrointestinal tract of man. *Gastroenterology* **45:** 721–729, 1963.

63. MacDonald, W. C., J. S. Trier, and N. B. Everett. Cell proliferation and migration in the stomach, duodenum and rectum of man: radioautographic studies. *Gastroenterology* **46:** 405–417, 1964.

64. McGuigan, J. E. Immunochemical studies with synthetic human gastrin. *Gastroenterology* **54:** 1005–1011, 1968.

65. Makhlouf, G. M., J. P. A. McManus, and W. I. Card. A comparative study of the effects of gastrin, histamine, histalog, and mechothane on the secretory capacity of the human stomach in two normal subjects over 20 months. *Gut* **6:** 525–534, 1965.

66. Makhlouf, G. M., J. P. A. McManus, and W. I. Card. A quantitative statement of the two-component hypothesis of gastric secretion. *Gastroenterology* **51:** 149–171, 1966.

67. Makhlouf, G. M., J. P. A. McManus, and W. I. Card. Comparative effects of gastrin II and histamine on pepsin secretion in man. *Gastroenterology* **52**: 787–791, 1967.

68. Makhlouf, G. M., J. P. A. McManus, and W. I. Card. The action of gastrin II on gastric secretion of electrolytes and pepsin in man. In: *Gastric Secretion: Mechanisms and Control*. Edited by T. K. Shnitka, J. A. L. Gilbert, and R. C. Harrison. New York: Pergamon Press, 1967, pp. 329–345.

69. Makhlouf, G. M., J. P. A. McManus, and J. R. Knill. Quantitative aspects of syngerism and inhibition of gastric acid secretion. *Gastroenterology* **54**: 532–537, 1968.

70. Meckeler, K. J. H. and F. J. Inglefinger. Correlation of electric surface potentials, intraluminal pressures, and nature of tissue in the gastroesophageal junction of man. *Gastroenterology* **52**: 966–971, 1967.

71. Menguy, R. Regulation of gastric mucus secretion. In: *Gastric Secretion: Mechanisms and Control*. Edited by T. K. Shnitka, J. A. L. Gilbert, and R. C. Harrison, New York: Pergamon Press, 1967, pp. 177–185.

72. Moody, F. G., and R. P. Durbin. Effects of glycine and other instillates on the concentration of gastric acid. *Am. J. Physiol.* **209**: 122–126, 1965.

73. Moody, F. G. Gastric blood flow and acid secretion during direct intra-arterial histamine administration. *Gastroenterology* **52**: 216–224, 1967.

74. Moore, E. W., and R. W. Scarlata. The determination of gastric acidity by the glass electrode. *Gastroenterology* **49**: 178–188, 1965.

75. Moore, E. W., T. L. Edwards, Jr., and J. F. Patterson. A mathematical method for estimation of maximal gastric secretory capacity. *Gastroenterology* **51**: 473–480, 1966.

76. Moore, E. W. Determination of pH by the glass electrode: pH meter calibration for gastric analysis. *Gastroenterology* **54**: 501–507, 1968.

77. Murphy, D. L., H. Goldstein, J. D. Boyle, and S. Ward. Hypercalcemia and gastric secretion in man. *J. Appl. Physiol.* **21**: 1607–1610, 1966.

78. Olbe, L. Vagal release of gastrin. In: *Gastrin*, edited by M. I. Grossman. Berkeley and Los Angeles: University of California Press, 1967, pp. 83–108.

79. Overholt, B. F., and H. M. Pollard, Acid diffusion into human gastric mucosa. *Gastroenterology* **54**: 182–189, 1968.

80. Penttila, A., and M. Lempinen. Enterochromaffin cells and 5-hydroxtryptamine in the human intestinal tract. *Gastroenterology* **54**: 375–381, 1968.

81. Piper, D. W., M. L. Macoun, J. E. Builder, and B. H. Fenton. Non-proteolytic enzymes in gastric juice. *Am. J. Dig. Dis.* **8**: 701–708, 1963.

82. Rune, S. J. Comparison of the rates of gastric acid secretion in man after ingestion of food and after maximal stimulation with histamine. *Gut* **7**: 344–350, 1966.

83. Rune, S. J. Proteolytic activity in the human stomach during digestion and its correlation with the augmented histamine test. *Gut* **7**: 69–72, 1966.

84. Schofield, B. Inhibition by acid of gastrin release. In: *Gastrin*, edited by M. I. Grossman, Berkeley and Los Angeles: University of California Press, 1967, pp. 171–192.

85. Schwartz, M., H. K. Kashiwa, A. Jacobson, and W. S. Rehm. Concentration and localization of calcium in frog gastric mucosa. *Am. J. Physiol.* **212**: 241–246, 1967.

86. Sedar, A. W. Fine structure of the stimulated oxyntic cell. *Fed. Proc.* **24**: 1360–1367, 1965.

87. Sircus, W. Prolonged augmentation of the maximal secretory responses of canine gastric pouches by chronic obstruction. *Am. J. Dig. Dis.* **10**: 499–505, 1965.

88. Smith, G. P., J. W. Mason, and E. D. Jacobson. Fasting gastric contents in conscious macaca mulatta. *Am. J. Physiol.* **211**: 629–633, 1966.

89. Smith, G. P., and P. R. McHugh. Gastric secretory response to amygdaloid or hypothalamic stimulation in monkeys. *Am. J. Physiol.* **213**: 640–644, 1967.

90. Smith, G. P., and F. P. Brooks. Hypothalamic control of gastric secretion. *Gastroenterology* **52**: 727–729, 1967.

91. Stoffels, G. L., W. Gepts, and J. J. Desneux. Histochemical study of the effect of enzyme inhibitors on gastric secretion. *Gut* **7**: 624–630, 1966.

92. Swan, K. G., and E. D. Jacobson. Gastric blood flow and secretion in conscious dogs. *Am. J. Physiol.* **212**: 891–896, 1967.

93. Sum, P. T., and R. M. Preshaw. Growth of the parietal cell population in the gastric mucosa of beagle dogs. *Gastroenterology* **54**: 1050–1056, 1968.

94. Turner, M. D., L. L. Miller, and H. L. Segal. Gastric proteases and protease inhibitors. *Gastroenterology* **53**: 967–983, 1967.

95. Villarreal, R. Pepsin secretion and synthesis in vitro. *Proc. Soc. Exp. Biol. Med.* **83**: 817–819, 1953.

96. Villegas, L. Cellular location of the electrical potential difference in frog gastric mucosa. *Biochim. Biophys. Acta* **64**: 359–367, 1962.

97. Villegas, L. Action of histamine on the permeability of the frog gastric mucosa to potassium and water. *Biochim. Biophys. Acta* **75**: 377–386, 1963.

98. Webster, D. R., E. W. Toovey, and S. C. Skoryna. Epithelial secretion of explanted gastric mucosa in rats. *Gastroenterology* **35**: 31–35, 1958.

99. Weir, D. G., I. J. Temperley, and D. Collery. Intrinsic factor secretion in response to continuous histamine infusion. *Gastroenterology* **52**: 23–28, 1967.

Additional Reading

Gastric Secretion. Mechanisms and Control, edited by T. K. Shnitka, J. A. L. Gilbert, and R. C. Harrison. New York: Pergamon Press, 1967.

Gastrin, edited by M. I. Grossman. Berkeley and Los Angeles: University of California Press, 1966.

Gregory, R. A. *Secretory Mechanisms of the Gastrointestinal Tract.* London: Edward Arnold & Co., 1962.

James, A. H. *The Physiology of Gastric Digestion.* London: Edward Arnold & Co., 1957.

Pathophysiology of Peptic Ulcer, edited by S. C. Skoryna. Philadelphia: J. B. Lippincott Co., 1963.

The Stomach, edited by C. M. Thompson, D. Berkowitz, and E. Polish. New York: Grune and Stratton. 1967.

CHAPTER

Pancreatic Secretion

THE EXOCRINE PORTION of the pancreas consists of a series of acini opening into ducts that eventually empty into the duodenum. Its principal products are sodium bicarbonate and enzymatic proteins. The mechanism for the secretion of sodium bicarbonate shares some of the properties of the system responsible for the secretion of hydrochloric acid by the stomach. The amount and variety of proteins made in the pancreas exceed those of the other digestive glands and make it a favorite organ for investigators studying protein synthesis.

Structural Basis for Pancreatic Secretion

The pancreas and the salivary glands, particularly the parotid, share many anatomic features. There is only one recognizable cell type in the acinus (88). This raises the interesting question of whether all cells are capable of synthesizing the whole variety of digestive enzymes, or whether there is specialization among cells. Using immunofluorescent techniques, Marshall found that individual acinar cells from bovine pancreas contained zymogen granules with both procarboxypeptidase and chymotrypsinogen; however, ribonuclease and deoxyribonuclease anitsera stained the cytoplasms of different cells (57). Yasuda and Koons used similar techniques in the pig pancreas and concluded that there was localization of specific enzymes within individual cells and that some secretory granules failed to fluoresce with any of the antisera used (105). Ehinger found that the mouse pancreas secreted ribonuclease by a mechanism partly independent of other proteins (24). It seems likely that there are specific areas specialized within individual cells for the synthesis of particular enzymes as well as a division of synthesis between cells.

Cytoplasmic inclusions without membranes or with only incomplete coats have been seen in the mouse pancreas (5) and in the rabbit (86). They may represent immature or maturing zymogen granules. Abe and his associates used histochemical techniques to demonstrate lipase in dog pancreatic acinar cells and found it concentrated in the Golgi region. They thought that lipase was probably outside the secretory granules (3). Enzyme secretion continues in the absence of secretory granules, which apparently represent a storage form.

In an attempt to correlate function with structure, Hansky et al. (32) related the maximal output of the canine pancreas to the weight of the gland in dogs. They found a generally linear relationship between maximal bicarbonate output after secretin and the weight of the gland, but this did not hold for the output of amylase after stimulation with pancreozymin and secretin.

Growth and Adaptation

Inhibitors of proteolytic enzyme activation produce an increase in the weight of the pancreas in several species (44,80). Hypertrophy was seen in the acini but not in the ducts (12). In chicks, pilocarpine failed to deplete tissue amylase, and there was an increase in the number of zymogen granules in the acinar cells (83). Geratz found that the enlargement of the rat pancreas induced by p-aminobezamidine was associated with an increase in tissue proteolytic enzymes but not amylase (27). He suggested that there may be stimulants acting on specific enzyme release and synthesis.

When protein-deficient animals were refed, there were hyperplasia and increased protein synthesis. While on a deficient diet, zymogen granules disappeared and the output of water, bicarbonate, and trypsin decreased. The changes reverted after two weeks on a normal diet (56).

Fitzgerald found that the pancreas had a regenerative capacity comparable to the liver in the rat (26). The evidence is not so convincing in man (92).

One of Pavlov's concepts was that the digestive glands had the capacity to adapt their secretion to the diet. The evidence for the salivary glands has been reviewed. Desnuelle and his colleagues in Marseilles have shown a threefold increase in amylase in the pancreas and in pancreatic secretion of rats fed a starch-rich diet (21,74). Similarly a casein-rich diet was followed by an increase in proteolytic enzymes (21,2). Digestion products of casein and starch were equally effective. The new levels of activity were reached within three to five days. Rats with alloxan diabetes have low levels of amylase which are restored with insulin (1). The blood sugar may serve as a signal to enzyme secretion. Adaptation involved a change in the number of enzyme molecules present in the pancreas and in pancreatic juice rather than a change in activity. Desnuelle calculated that on a starch diet, the rat pancreas could synthesize 2.4 $\times$ 10^6 amylase molecules/minute and 5.2 $\times$ 10^5 chymotrypsin molecules (20). Other workers found that adaptation occurred after vagotomy in rats, excluding a vagal mechanism (59).

Some Properties of the Pancreas

The electrical properties of the pancreas are now being studied in much the same way that the salivary glands had been examined earlier. Clark and his colleagues (16) studied conductance and capacitance across the pancreas in cat. After stimulation with secretin, there was a brief increase in conductance followed by a more marked decrease. The latter phase correlated with the flow of pancreatic juice. The authors suggested that it might be due to swelling of the secretory cells.

Dean and Matthews recorded intracellular potentials in mouse pancreatic acinar cells (17). They found resting potentials of -41 mv. They also observed spontaneous miniature depolarization potentials of 0.5 to 2.5 mv. These were decreased by atropine. Physostigmine, an anticholinesterase, was followed by an increase in the amplitude and frequency of the miniature potentials. Nerve stimulation produced depolarization of acinar cells, as did cholinergic drugs. These effects were blocked by atropine. They suggested that depolarization by nerve stimulation may trigger secretion.

Little is known of the permeability characteristics of the pancreatic ducts. Dreiling and his colleagues perfused the major duct from the tail to the head of the pancreas in dogs with a solution containing 154 mEq/L of bicarbonate. In each experiment bicarbonate left the ducts (96).

Methods of Study

Pure pancreatic secretion can be obtained only through catheterization of the pancreatic ducts. In animals the pancreatic duct and a surrounding cuff of duodenal mucosa can be brought out on the surface of the abdomen. The proteolytic enzymes collected from the duct will be inactive. For example, trypsinogen must be converted to trypsin by an enzyme from the intestinal mucosa, enterokinase, or by trypsin itself. Amylase is fully active and lipase is partially active.

In man, pancreatic secretion is studied by passing a double-lumen tube into the duodenum and positioning it in such a fashion that gastric content can be aspirated separately from duodenal content. Pancreatic secretion can then be stimulated by the administration of humoral or parasympathomimetic agents. It is likely that as much as 20 per cent of duodenal fluid may escape into the jejunum under these conditions (55).

Composition of Pancreatic Secretion

WATER AND ELECTROLYTES

As in the case of the salivary glands and the stomach, the electrolyte composition of pancreatic juice varies with the rate of secretion. Figure 5-1 shows the relationship of bicarbonate, chloride, sodium, and potassium concentrations to flow. Banwell et al. found the maximum bicarbonate concentration in man after a continuous infusion of secretin to be 124 to 127 mEq/L (6). Sodium and potassium are present in concentrations approximating those in plasma. In dogs the concentration of calcium in pancreatic juice was found to be less than that in plasma and possibly related to the digestive enzymes. Calcium may be part of the amylase molecule (106).

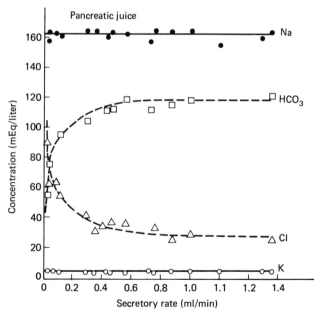

FIGURE 5-1 Graphs to show the relationship between the electrolyte concentrations in pancreatic juice and the volume secreted. (From F. Bro-Rasmussen, J. H. Thaysen, and S. A. Killman. *Acta Physiol. Scand.,* **37:** 97, 1956.)

The pancreas produces a bewildering menage of proteins, most of them enzymes. Keller and Allan reported the following from human pancreatic secretion: lipase, ribonuclease, deoxyribonuclease, proelastase, procarboxy-peptidases A and B, chymotrypsinogen, trypsinogen, and trypsin inhibitor (49). Greene et al. found the trypsin inhibitor of bovine pancreatic juice to be a polypeptide with a molecular weight of 6,155 (29). It was present in a concentration of 0.6 mg/Gm of protein. It prevents the activation of the zymogen by trypsin.

The concentration of pancreatic enzymes is expressed most satisfactorily in terms of micromoles of substrate split per unit time. This is possible with synthetic substrates such as those available for trypsin and chymotrypsin. Amylase, however, is usually assayed by colorimetric measurement of reducing sugars and expressed in terms of units.

Pancreatic amylase is an alpha amylase. The question of isoamylases is still under study. Trypsin and chymotrypsin are endopeptidases which split the peptide bonds within the molecule, while carboxypeptidases are exo-peptidases acting only on the terminal peptide bonds.

Since measurement of individual pancreatic enzymes is laborious, some workers have taken advantage of the fact that most of the protein in pancreatic juice is enzymatic to use measurements of total protein as an indicator of enzyme content (31).

Babkin proposed that pancreatic enzymes were secreted in parallel concentrations. If true, this would permit measurement of a single enzyme as representative of all. Unfortunately this is probably not the case (81).

Stimulation of secretion to maximal levels is usually associated with less variability than resting secretion. As stimulants such as secretin and pancreo-zymin become available in pure form, stimulation at the plateau of a dose-response curve becomes feasible. Stimulation by continuous infusion provides a steady state, if other factors do not reduce secretory capacity. In man, Banwell et al. found that the variability for the rate of secretion and bicarbonate output could be reduced further by expressing results in terms of body weight. However, the maximum amylase output after pancreozymin was independent of body weight (7). Wormsley reported that the volume of duodenal content recovered after maximal continuous stimulation with secretin in man was inversely related to the bicarbonate concentration, while the chloride concentration and sodium output were linearly related to the volume (103). Figure 5-2 illustrates his results.

Pancreatic secretion also contains a small amount of mucus. Little is known of the characteristics of this material in comparison to mucus elsewhere in the digestive tract. Small amounts of serum proteins can also be detected in pancreatic juice.

Mechanisms of Pancreatic Secretion

ELECTROLYTES

By analogy with the stomach, the relàtionships between bicarbonate and chloride in pancreatic juice have been explained by a two-component or admixture hypothesis. The acini were assumed to elaborate a secretion high in bicarbonate concentration which was diluted by a chloride secretion in the ducts, especially at low rates of flow. More recently, by analogy with the kidney, an ion exchange hypothesis has been suggested with an exchange of bicarbonate for chloride taking place in the ducts. Finally there remains a unicellular hypothesis with a single cell having the capability of varying the composition of its output.

There is no direct resolution of these conflicting theories. Recently Reber and Wolf were able to obtain samples from the ducts just external to the intercalated ducts in rabbits and found that the composition of secretion at slow and rapid rates of flow was the same in the small ducts as in the major duct (73). Stop-flow techniques have failed to identify the site of a bicarbonate-chloride exchange in the dog.

The bicarbonate of pancreatic secretion is derived in part from the plasma and to some extent from endogenous metabolism within the pancreas (47). Whether transport occurs as bicarbonate or as CO_2 is unknown. The gradient influencing movement could be either pCO_2 or bicarbonate concentration. With the in vitro pancreas, the pCO_2 of pancreatic juice relative to that of the bath rose as the temperature of the bath was increased (42).

The enzyme carbonic anhydrase is present in the pancreas. Histochemical studies localize the activity to the ductal cells (8). Acetazolamide inhibits pancreatic secretion (23). However, as in the stomach, the evidence does not implicate the enzyme directly in the formation of bicarbonate.

Metabolic alkalosis favors the secretion of bicarbonate, and acetazolamide reverses the effect. Metabolic and respiratory acidosis hinder secretion (63,72).

Removal of sodium, chloride, and bicarbonate and replacement with appropriate substitutes in the bath result in marked reduction in secretory rate by the in vitro pancreas (76). These results are compatible with a "unicellular" theory.

Debray et al. found that isotopes of Na and K given intravenously to man appeared promptly in pancreatic juice and reached peak activities in about 30 minutes (18).

Henriksen and Worning found that the relationship between bicarbonate and protein concentrations in pancreatic juice from dogs after feeding was a straight line, favoring the admixture theory (36). Stop-flow studies in dogs showed a fall in bicarbonate concentration and a rise in chloride, as might

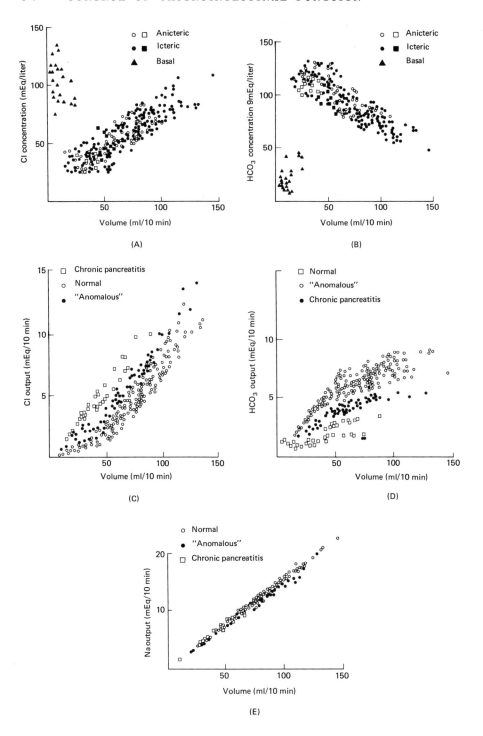

be expected with a bicarbonate-chloride exchange, but unfortunately not in the same samples (66).

There remains agreement that the secretion of bicarbonate is an energy-requiring process (75).

PROTEINS

The mechanisms of protein synthesis and secretion are known largely through a combination of morphologic and biochemical studies (64). The distinction between secretion or extrusion and synthesis must be emphasized. Current models of the cellular machinery of enzyme synthesis and secretion picture events as follows: Complementary messenger RNA is formed on DNA in the nucleus. It leaves the nucleus and attaches to the ribosomes. Other RNA molecules, transfer RNA, carrying specific amino acids, attach in a complementary manner to the messenger RNA on the ribosomes. With the arrival of the next transfer RNA molecule, the amino acids form a peptide linkage, and the first transfer RNA molecule falls away, leaving the dipeptide attached to the ribosome by the second transfer RNA molecule. In this fashion, the complete polypeptide is assembled when the last transfer RNA molecule falls away from the last portion of the messenger RNA molecule. The linkage between messenger RNA and transfer RNA is thought to consist of triplets of nucleotides in complementary fashion. Each triplet of nucleotides is specific for an amino acid, but most amino acids are represented by more than one triplet. Figure 5-3 illustrates the concept.

Beeley et al. have purified canine pancreatic ribosomes and found them to contain 60 per cent RNA (9). They found 21 cationic components in the protein moiety (50). Some were species specific. The antibiotic tetracycline inhibited the specific binding of phenylalanine transfer RNA to ribosomes (90).

Once assembled on the ribosomes, the enzymatic proteins are thought

FIGURE   5-2   A. Normal relationship of chloride concentration to volume of duodenal aspirate. Significance of points as in B. B: Normal relationship of bicarbonate concentration to volume of duodenal aspirate. Each point represents the bicarbonate concentration and volume of one 10-min sample of duodenal aspirate form normal subjects and patients with duodenal ulcer or gallstones. Each subject contributed 2 to 4 points during different levels of secretin stimulation; o and •, values during the steady state response to secretin infusions; □ and ■, samples taken during the second 10-min period after secretin injections; o and □, samples free from bile pigment; • and ■, bile-stained samples. C: Relationship to chloride output to volume of duodenal aspirate. Significance of points as in D. D: Relationship of bicarbonate output to volume of duodenal aspirate. Each point represents one (or a group of) value (s) of bicarbonate output and the volume of the appropriate sample, during the 10-min collection period, during the steady state response to secretin infusions. Vertical bars through the points indicate samples free of bile pigment. E: Relationship of sodium output to volume of duodenal aspirate. Significance of the points as in D. (From K. G. Wormsley. *Gastroenterology* **54:** 197–209, © 1968, The Williams & Wilkens Co., Baltimore, Md. 21202, U.S.A.)

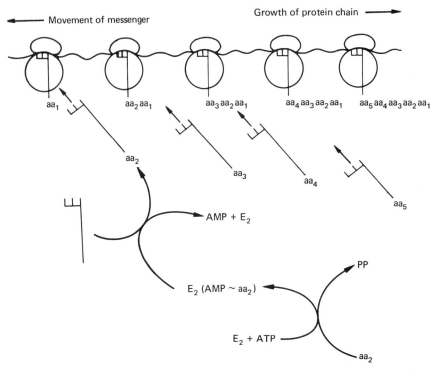

FIGURE 5-3. Scheme of protein synthesis including amino acid activation, attachment of amino acid to sRNA and transfer of amino acids to protein in ribosomes. Five ribosomes are shown threaded with their messenger. Transfer RNA molecules are three-pronged at one end to represent three nucleotides which recognize the codon on the messenger (sometimes called the "nodoc"!). (From M. B. Hoagland. In J. B. Stanbury et al. *Metabolic Bases of Inherited Diseases.* New York: McGraw-Hill, 1960.)

to begin a journey through the tubular system of the endoplasmic reticulum to the Golgi apparatus. Here the membrane of the zymogen granule is added, and the secretory granule moves to the apex of the cell. At the luminal surface the membrane of the zymogen granule fuses with the cell membrane, and the zymogen is released into the lumen (45,46).

Siekevitz and Palade reported that certain of the cisternae of the endoplasmic reticulum were exclusively or predominantly engaged in amylase production, while possibly others were responsible for the synthesis of other enzymes (87).

Hokin has made extensive studies of the role of phospholipids in the secretion of pancreatic enzymes (41). They suggest that the enzymatic protein in the cisternae of the endoplasmic reticulum is incorporated into a zymogen granule by budding off of membranes from the Golgi apparatus or by enlargement of vesicles by formation of new membranes.

The incorporation of amino acids into digestive enzymes can be studied by using isotopically labeled amino acids. It takes about one or two minutes to synthesize a digestive enzyme and about an hour for it to appear in pancreatic juice (41). When ^{35}S-labeled methionine was given to humans, with catheters in the pancreas, the peak specific activity in pancreatic juice was reached in eight hours and exceeded that in the serum by a factor of nine to one (53). The half-life in pancreatic juice was three days. After the intravenous administration of selenomethionine to dogs, the labeled sulfur appeared in pancreatic juice in significant quantities in one hour, almost exclusively in the protein fraction precipitated by trichloracetic acid (93). This is consistent with the time required for synthesis and extrusion of zymogen granules reported by others (95). They found that the life-span of a zymogen granule was 48 minutes. Begin and Scholefield found that the uptake of glycine by mouse pancreas in vitro was inhibited by dinitrophenol and when sodium chloride in the medium was replaced by choline chloride. Absence of potassium and the addition of ouabain also inhibited uptake (10).

Control of Pancreatic Secretion

CELLULAR CONTROL

The effects of parasympathomimetic drugs and pancreozymin on the extrusion and synthesis of pancreatic enzymes have been studied in intact animals, in virtro pancreas, and especially pigeon pancreas slices. All agree that extrusion of enzymes result. However, there is disagreement over the effects on enzyme synthesis. Hokin and Hokin found that acetylcholine or pancreozymin caused a burst of labeling of phosphatidyl inositol with ^{32}P (39). The effect occurred in microsomes on both smooth-and rough-surfaced membranes and may represent a general effect on the transmembrane transport of zymogens. There was an increased grain density over the cytoplasm of acinar cells but not over the nuclei (40). It was localized to tissue lipid. The Golgi apparatus and rough-surfaced endoplasmic reticulum were considered to be independent sites of the increase in synthesis of phospholipid. There was no evidence of increased synthesis of enzymes. On the other hand, Webster and Tyor found that pancreatic slices from pigeons given pancreozymin intravenously incorporated phenylalanine into protein at a faster rate 60 to 120 minutes after giving the hormone (99). After feeding, there was an increased incorporation of uridine-^{3}H into RNA in pancreas slices (101). Similarly, feeding increased fatty acid oxidation and the incorporation of palmitate into triglyceride and fatty acid (98,100). Peakall found an increased rate of synthesis of DNA and of protein in the first hour after cholinergic stimulation of pigeons (65). He considered that an increased secretory rate signaled increased synthesis. Webster also found an increase in uridine-^{3}H incorporation into pigeon pancreas slices after methacholine (*102*). This could be blocked by prior administration of actinomycin D. The increase in incorporation of phenylalanine into protein was only partially blocked by actinomycin D. Acetylcholine may act on cell genomes to induce messenger RNA synthesis.

In the rat, Kramer and Poort found that pilocarpine caused the discharge of zymogen granules but failed to increase protein synthesis. They concluded that the protein synthetic rate was constant and uninfluenced by extrusion of enzyme (*51*). Rothman made similar observations in rabbits but found a nonparallel transport of enzymes after pancreozymin, while methacholine increased output of both trypsinogen and chymotrypsinogen in pancreatic juice (*77*).

In longer-term experiments, pancreozymin given to rats increased the weight of the pancreas and produced hypertrophy of acinar cells. Secretin and methacholine did not (*78*).

HORMONAL CONTROL

This subject has been clarified by the purification of secretin and pancreozymin and the synthesis of secretin (*33*). Secretin is a polypeptide consisting of 27 amino acids with a sequence resembling glucagon, as shown in Figure 5-4(A) (*60*). Subsequently an equally potent synthetic product has been prepared (*11*). No physiologic activity was obtained starting from the C-terminal end of the molecule until the peptide 2-27 was reached. Adding histidine increased the activity more than a hundredfold. Starting at the amino end gave some activity after the first 13 residues. The two biologic activities known as pancreozymin and cholecystokinin are now known to reside in a single polypeptide. It consists of 33 amino acids and has the same C-terminal tetrapeptide as gastrin (*61*). Figure 5-4 (B) shows the structure of the physiologically active octapeptide. These great accomplishments have made it possible to express dosage in unit of weight rather than biologic activity and have settled the vexing problem of contaminants. The structure of gastrin has already been reviewed.

Both secretin and pancreozymin are present in extracts of small intestinal mucosa. Clifton and his colleagues found secretin activity in dogs confined to the villi (*52*). They concluded that secretin must reside in the stroma of the villi or the villous epithelial cells. Little is known of the cellular origin of pancreozymin.

The mechanism of action of these hormones on the pancreas is unknown. Secretin acts primarily to increase the output of water and bicarbonate (*62*). When given in the perfusing fluid to isolated dog pancreas, the only structural change was the presence of a few pinocytotic vesicles in the ductal margin of the intercalated duct cells (*43*).

Pancreozymin acts primarily to increase the output of enzyme from the pancreas. In the perfused dog pancreas there is an increased output of pro-

Secretin: *His*· *Ser*· Asp· *Gly*· *Thr*· *Phe*· *Thr*· Ser·
Glu· Leu· *Ser*· Arg· Leu· Arg· *Asp*· Ser· Ala· *Arg*·
Leu· *Gln*· Arg· Leu· Leu· *Gln*· Gly· *Leu*· Val· NH₂

Glucagon: *His*· Ser· Gln· *Gly*· Thr· Phe· Thr· Ser·
Asp· Tyr· Ser· Lys· Tyr· Leu· *Asp*· Ser· Arg· Arg·
Ala· *Gln*· Asp· Phe· Val· *Gln*· Try· *Leu*· Met· Asn· Thr

(A)

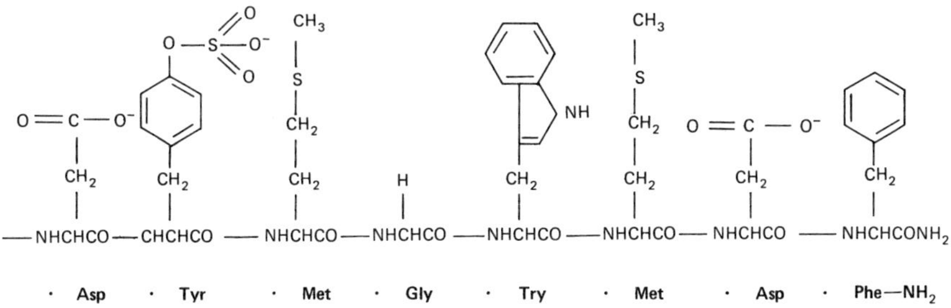

· Asp · Tyr · Met · Gly · Try · Met · Asp · Phe—NH₂

(B)

FIGURE 5-4.   A: Amino acid sequences of secretin and glucagon. B: The C-terminal octapeptide of cholecystokinin. (From J. E. Jorpes. *Gastroenterology* **55**: 163, © 1968, The Williams & Wilkins Co., Baltimore, Md. 21202, U.S.A.)

tein and a depletion of zymogen granules (*43*). Case and his associates found that the osmolarity of pancreatic juice during secretin stimulation from the perfused cat pancreas mirrored that of the perfusate. They offered two hypotheses—that the pancreas secretes a primary bicarbonate secretion modified by exchange across the ducts, with the primary secretion depressed by changes in the osmolarity and NaCl concentration of the perfusate, or that the primary pancreatic secretion always had the same osmolarity as the perfusate.

Gastrin also acts primarily to increase the protein output of the pancreas. Gastrin I in amounts approaching maximal gastric stimulation caused a threefold increase in protein output in dogs (*67*).

Henriksen and Worning reported potentiation of the secretin-induced output of bicarbonate from the pancreas in dogs by pancreozymin, but the effect on protein secretion was only additive (*37*).

The importance of secretin and pancreozymin in the control of pancreatic secretion in vivo is illustrated by the fact that a transplanted and hence denervated portion of the pancreas in dogs responded to a variety of stimuli, including peptides, fats, and sugars, in a qualitatively similar fashion to the intact pancreas (*94*).

The control of the release of secretin from the intestinal mucosa is similar to that of gastrin release from the antrum. Here, however, the release appears to be proportional to the amount of hydrogen ion entering the duodenum rather than the hydrogen ion concentration (*70*). It is of some interest that, in the dog, the amount of HCl produced in response to a meal exceeds that of bicarbonate by a factor of 6:1 (79). In man, submaximal secretin stimulation produced as much bicarbonate as maximal acid secretion did H^+ (4).

NEURAL CONTROL

The evidence for neural control of pancreatic secretion rests largely on the effects of blocking or stimulating the vagi and the influence of cholinergic or anticholinergic drugs (91). Harper and his associates showed that electrical stimulation of the cut central end of the vagus in the cat sometimes increased amylase output from the pancreas, provided the opposite vagus was intact. Stimulation of efferent fibers in the vagus regularly increased amylase output (34). Thomas found that the excitatory effect of peptone in the duodenum was temporarily abolished by vagotomy (91), and Magee and White reported a similar effect on the response to distention of the fundus of the stomach, a "gastropancreatic reflex" (97). The cytologic correlate of this reflex in the frog was reported to be an increase in the number of secretory granules per acinar cell (58).

Blocking the vagi in the neck in conscious dogs resulted in an abrupt decrease in pancreatic secretion in response to intraduodenal peptone. In all of these experiments the neural effect was largely upon enzyme output rather than water and electrolyte. No permanent defect in response to stimulation has been demonstrated after vagotomy (91).

Anticholinergic drugs block the action of secretin on pancreatic secretion and the effect of HCl in the duodenum. Recent dose-response studies suggest that the latter is more susceptible to inhibition (84). The release of secretin in response to HCl can be inhibited by a topical anesthetic, reminiscent of the control of gastrin release from the antrum (89). However, the details are not as well understood. Junqueira et al. found that atropine inhibited release of zymogen granules without effect on synthesis (48).

Sympathetic effects on pancreatic secretion are difficult to dissociate from effects on blood flow. No sympathetic fibers have been demonstrated in close association with acinar cells. Greenwell and his colleagues stimulated the cut peripheral end of a splanchnic nerve in anesthetized cats and found an increase in amylase output in spite of a coincident decrease in blood flow and volume secretion (30). Atropine selectively blocked the increase in amylase output, suggesting it was mediated by cholinergic fibers in the sympathetics.

In man, Sarles et al. demonstrated a clear-cut cephalic phase of pancreatic secretion in response to sham feeding. Volume, bicarbonate output, and enzyme secretion all increased (82). However, Dreiling et al. could find no change in the secretory response to secretin after vagotomy in man (22). Insulin hypoglycemia stimulated pancreatic secretion in man and dogs, presumably by a vagal mechanism (13,25). There is some evidence that the hypothalamus may influence duodenal sphincter tone and indirectly alter the pancreatic secretory rate (28).

GASTRIC PHASE

Preshaw demonstrated that acetylcholine perfusion of an antral pouch increased protein output from a transplanted pancreas and that this could be blocked by acidifying the antrum (68,71). He and his associates also showed that sham feeding increased pancreatic protein secretion and that this could be inhibited by acidifying the antrum (69). These observations suggest that some vagal and antral effects on pancreatic secretion may be mediated by the release of gastrin.

RELATIONSHIPS BETWEEN STIMULI

The complex interactions between hormones and between humoral and neural stimuli are difficult to interpret. Species differences must be considered. In dogs, Henriksen found that secretin and pancreozymin together were more potent stimulants of fluid and bicarbonate than secretin alone (38). In three of four dogs the combination of the two hormones gave greater protein outputs than pancreozymin alone. Wormsley found that continuous infusions of secretin in man increased trypsin output at low doses and inhibited it at high doses (104). With prolonged secretin infusions, lipase activity may disappear.

EXTRAINTESTINAL HORMONAL CONTROL

Little is known of the relationships of the other endocrine glands to the pancreas. Sesso et al. found that thyroxin increased both synthesis and extrusion of amylase in hypophysectomized rats, while cortisone increased synthesis only (85). The clinical observation of the association between pancreatitis and hyperparathyroidism is unexplained.

BLOOD FLOW AND SECRETION

Using anesthetized dogs, Delaney and Grim found pancreatic blood flow to be increased by secretin and little changed by pancreozymin (19). However, in a study of the microcirculation of the pancreas in rabbits, pancreozymin (cecekin) produced vasodilation and increased flow (35). Vagal stimulation upon a background of secretin infusion in cats increased output of amylase and the concentration of bicarbonate (14). Pancreozymin, antral extracts, and histamine under similar circumstances increased flow and amylase output. The common factor may be an increase in blood flow with a delivery of more secretin to the secreting cells.

Function of the Pancreas in Man

The main role of the pancreas in man is in the elaboration and secretion of digestive enzymes. Total pancreatectomy results in excessive amounts of fat in the stools and in increased nitrogen loss. In pancreatic disease the steatorrhea usually is the dominant defect. Bicarbonate secretion may be important in the control of duodenal pH, both as a protection against gastric HCl and to maintain an optimum environment for the digestive enzymes of the small intestine.

Pathophysiology

As in the stomach, secretory rest of an inflamed pancreas seems to be desirable, although evidence is inconclusive (54). Draining the stomach and the administration of anticholinergic drugs might be expected to reduce pancreatic secretion. The steatorrhea of pancreatic insufficiency can be partially corrected by the administration of pancreatic enzymes.

Summary

The exocrine pancreas is composed of acinar cells, which exhibit active protein synthesis of enzymes, and ductal cells, which may have secretory and absorptive functions for water and electrolyte. It is likely that there is specialization within cells and between acinar cells for the synthesis of specific proteins. Therefore the enzyme response to stimuli will vary in proportion to specific enzymes. Adaptation of enzyme secretion to diet occurs rapidly and independently of neural control. Hormonal control of secretion dominates the pancreas. Transplanted pancreas responds to dietary and humoral stimuli in a qualitatively normal fashion. Secretin stimulates water and bicarbonate secretion, while pancreozymin and gastrin act primarily upon enzyme output. Vagal stimulation also acts on enzyme output and may act indirectly by the release of gastrin. The rudiments of an autoregulatory system for the control of pancreatic secretion exist. Secretin release depends upon the amount of HCl in the duodenum, and bicarbonate reduces the amount of hydrgen ion. There may be a cholinergic nervous arc involved in secretin release. The similar C-terminal tetrapeptide in gastrin and pancreozymin suggests some similarity in function.

References

1. Abdeljlil, A. B., J. C. Palla, and P. Desnuelle. Effect of insulin on pancreatic amylase and chymotrypsinogen. *Biochem. Biophys. Res. Commun.* **18**: 71–75, 1965.
2. Abdeljlil, A. B. Adaptation of the enzymes of exocrine pancreas in response to alimentary and hormonal stimuli. *Gut* **7**: 298, 1966.
3. Abe, M., S. P. Kramer, and A. M. Seligman. The histochemical demonstration of pancreatic-like lipase and comparison with the distribution of esterase. *J. Histochem. Cytochem.* **12**: 364–383, 1964.

4. Banks, P. A., W. P. Dyck, D. A. Dreiling, and H. D. Janowitz. Secretory capacity of stomach and pancreas in man. *Gastroenterology* **53**: 575–578, 1967.

5. Bannasch, P. Hullenlose Cytoplasmaininclusionen und ihre Beziehung zur Sekretbildung in exokrinen Pancreas der Maus. *J. Ultrastruct. Res.* **15**: 528–542, 1966.

6. Banwell, G., B. E. Northam, and W. T. Cooke. Secretory response of the human pancreas to continuous intravenous infusion of secretin. *Gut* **8**: 50–57, 1967.

7. Banwell, J. G., B. E. Northam, and W. T. Cooke. Secretory response of the human pancreas to continuous intravenous infusion of pancreozymincholecystokinin (Cecekin). *Gut* **8**: 380–387, 1967.

8. Becker, V. Histochemistry of the exocrine pancreas. In: *The Exocrine Pancreas.* Edited by A. V. S. de Reuck and M. P. Cameron. Boston: Little, Brown & Co., 1962, pp. 56–63.

9. Beeley, J. A. H., E. Cohen, and P. J. Keller. Canine pancreatic ribosomes. *J. Biol. Chem.* **243**: 1262–1270, 1968.

10. Begin, N., and P. G. Scholefield. The uptake of amino acids by mouse pancreas in vitro. *Biochim. Biophys. Acta.* **90**: 82–89, 1964.

11. Bodansky, M., M. A. Ondetti, S. D. Levine, V. L. Narayanan, M. von Salzta, J. T. Sheehan, N. J. Williams, and E. F. Sabo. Synthesis of a heptacosapeptide amide with the hormonal activity of secretin. *Chem. Industr.* **42**: 1757–1758, 1966.

12. Booth, A. N., D. J. Robbins, W. E. Ribelin, F. DeEds, A. K. Smith, and J. J. Rackis. Prolonged pancreatic hypertrophy and reversibility in rats fed raw soybean meal. *Proc. Soc. Exp. Biol. Med.* **116**: 1067–1069, 1964.

13. Brooks, F. P., and H. Manfredo. The control of pancreatic secretion and its clinical significance. *Am. J. Gastroenterol.* **42**: 42–46, 1964.

14. Brown, J. C., A. A. Harper, and T. Scratcherd. Potentiation of secretin stimulation of the pancreas. *J. Physiol. London* **190**: 519–530, 1967.

15. Case, R. M., A. A. Harper, and T. Scratcherd. Water and electrolyte secretion by the perfused pancreas of the cat. *J. Physiol. London* **196**: 133–149, 1968.

16. Clark, D. G., J. R. Greenwell, A. A. Harper, A. M. Sankey, and T. Scratcherd. The electrical properties of resting and secreting pancreas. *J. Physiol. London* **189**: 247–260, 1967.

17. Dean, P. M., and E. K. Matthews. Miniature depolarization potentials in pancreatic acinar cells. *Proc. Physiol. Soc.*, July 1968, pp. 37–38.

18. Debray, C., M. Roux, C. Sautier, J. Tremolieres, and J. P. Hardouin, Etude de la secretion pancreatique chez l'homme a l'aide de radioelements Na^{24} et K^{42}. *Rev. Franc. Etud. Clin. Biol.* **9**: 516–517, 1964.

19. Delaney, J. P., and E. Grim. Influence of hormones and drugs on canine pancreatic blood flow. *Am. J. Physiol.* **211**: 1398–1402, 1966.

20. Desnuelle, P. Adaptation of the enzymes of exocrine pancreas in terms of biosynthesis. *Gut* **7**: 298–299, 1966.

21. Desnuelle, P., J. P. Reboud, and A. B. Abdeljlil. Influence of the compositon of the diet on the enzyme content of the rat pancreas. In: *The Exocrine Pancreas.* Edited by A. V. S. de Reuck and M. P. Cameron. Boston: Little, Brown & Co., 1962, pp. 90–114.

22. Dreiling, D. A., L. J. Druckerman, and F. Hollander. The effect of complete

vagisection and vagal stimulation on pancreatic secretion in man. *Gastroenterol ogy* **20:** 578–586, 1952.

23. Dreiling, D. A., H. D. Janowitz, and M. Halpern. The effect of a carbonic anhydrase inhibitor, diamox, on human pancreatic secretion. *Gastroenterology* **29:** 262–279, 1955.

24. Ehinger, B. On the mechanism of ribonuclease secretion in the murine exocrine pancreas. *Histochemie* **5:** 326–330, 1965.

25. Eisenberg, M. M., and M. I. Grossman. Pancreatic exocrine response to 2-deoxy-D-glucose, insulin and histamine. *Surg. Forum* **17:** 349–351, 1966.

26. Fitzgerald, P. J., B. M. Carol, and L. Rosenstock. Pancreatic acinar cell regeneration. *Nature* **212:** 594–596, 1966.

27. Geratz, J. D. Growth retardation and pancreatic enlargement in rats due to p-aminobenzamidine. *Am. J. Physiol.* **214:** 595–600, 1968.

28. Gilsdorf, R. B., J. M. Pearl, and A. S. Leonard. Central autonomic influences on pancreatic duct pressure and secretory rates. *Surg. Forum* **17:** 341–342, 1966.

29. Greene, L. J., M. Rigbi, and D. S. Fackre. Trypsin inhibitor from bovine pancreatic juice. *J. Biol. Chem.* **241:** 5610–5618, 1966.

30. Greenwell, R., A. A. Harper, and T. Scratcherd. Effects of splanchnic nerve stimulation on pancreatic secretion, blood flow and electrical conductance. *Gut* **8:** 635, 1967.

31. Hanscom, H. D., B. M. Jacobson, and A. Littman. The output of protein after pancreozymin. A test of pancreatic function. *Ann. Intern. Med.* **66:** 721–726, 1967.

32. Hansky, J., O. M. Tiscornia, D. A. Dreiling, and H. D. Janowitz. Relationship between maximal secretory output and weight of the pancreas in the dog. *Proc. Soc. Exp. Biol. Med.* **114:** 654–656, 1963.

33. Harper, A. A. Hormonal control of pancreatic secretion. In: *Handbook of Physiology.* Section 6: Alimentary Tract. Vol. II: Secretion. Edited by C. F. Code. Washington D.C.: American Physiological Society, 1967, pp. 969–995.

34. Harper, A. A., C. Kidd, and T. Scratcherd. Vago-vagal reflex effects on gastric and pancreatic secretion and gastrointestinal motility. *J. Physiol. London* **148:** 417–436, 1959.

35. Heisig, N. Pancreatic microcirculation under the influence of adequate secretory stimulation. *Bibl. Anat.* **9:** 176–180, 1967.

36. Henriksen, F. W., and H. Worning. The relation between the concentrations of bicarbonate and protein in the pancreatic juice in the dog. *J. Physiol. London* **187:** 285–289, 1966.

37. Henriksen, F. W., and H. Worning. The interaction of secretin and pancreozymin on the external pancreatic secretion in dogs, *Acta Physiol. Scand.* **70:** 241–249, 1967.

38. Henriksen, F. W. The maximal pancreatic secretion in dogs. *Scand. J. Gastroenterol.* **3:** 140–144, 1968.

39. Hokin, L. E., and M. R. Hokin. Changes in phospholipid metabolism on stimulation of protein secretion in pancreas slices. *J. Histochem. Cytochem.* **13:** 113–116, 1965.

40. Hokin, L. E., and D. Huebner. Radioautographic localization of increased synthesis of phosphatidylinositol in response to pancreozymin or acetylcholine in guinea pig pancreas slices. *J. Cell. Biol.* **33:** 521–530, 1967.

41. Hokin, L. E. Metabolic aspects and energetics of pancreatic secretion. In: *Handbook of Physiology*. Section 6: Alimentary Tract. Vol. II: Secretion. Edited by C. F. Code. Washington D.C.: American Physiological Society, 1967, pp. 935–953.

42. Hubel, K. A. In vitro rabbit pancreas: Effect of temperature on HCO_3, PCO_2, pH and flow. *Am. J. Physiol.* **212:** 101–103, 1967.

43. Ichikawa, A. Fine structural changes in response to hormonal stimulation of perfused canine pancreas. *J. Cell. Biol.* **24:** 369–385, 1965.

44. Imondi, A. R., and F. H. Bird. Effects of dietary protein level on growth and proteolytic activity of the avian pancreas. *J. Nutr.* **91:** 421–428, 1967.

45. Jamieson, J. D., and G. E. Palade. Intracellular transport of secretory proteins in the pancreatic acinar cell. I. Role of the peripheral elements of the Golgi apparatus. *J. Cell. Biol.* **34:** 577–596, 1967.

46. Jamieson, J. D., and G. E. Palade. Intracellular transport of secretory proteins in the pancreatic exocrine cell. II. Transport to condensing vacuoles and zymogen granules. *J. Cell. Biol.* **34:** 597–615, 1967.

47. Janowitz, H. D. Pancreatic secretion of fluid and electrolytes. In: *Handbook of Physiology*. Section 6: Alimentary Tract. Vol. II: Secretion. Edited by C. F. Code. Washington D. C.: American Physiological Society, 1967, pp. 925–933.

48. Junqueira, L. C. U., H. A. Rothchild, and I. Vugman. The action of atropine on pancreatic secretion. *Brit. J. Pharmacol.* **13:** 71–73, 1958.

49. Keller, P. J., and B. J. Allan. The protein composition of human pancreatic juice. *J. Biol. Chem.* **242:** 281–287, 1967.

50. Keller, P. J., E. Cohen, and J. A. H. Beely. Canine pancreatic ribosomes. II. The protein moiety. *J. Biol. Chem.* **243:** 1271–1276, 1968.

51. Kramer, M. F., and C. Poort. Protein synthesis in the pancreas of the rat after stimulation of secretion. *Z. Zellforsch.* **86:** 475–486, 1968.

52. Krawitt, E. L., G. R. Zimmerman, and J. A. Clifton. Localization of secretin in dog duodenal mucosa. *Am. J. Physiol.* **211:** 935–938, 1966.

53. Kukral, J. C., A. P. Adams, and F. W. Preston. Protein producing capacity of the human exocrine pancreas: Incorporation of S^{35} methionine in serum and pancreatic juice protein. *Ann. Surg.* **162:** 63–73, 1965.

54. Lagerlof, H. D. Pancreatic secretion: pathophysiology. In: *Handbook of Physiology*. Section 6: Alimentary Tract. Vol. II: Secretion. Edited by C. F. Code. Washington D.C.: American Physiological Society, 1967, pp. 1027–1042.

55. Lagerlof, H. D., H. B. Schutz, and S. Holmer. A secretin test with high doses of secretin and correction for incomplete recovery of duodenal juice. *Gastroenterology* **52:** 67–77, 1967.

56. Lemire, S., and F. L. Iber. Pancreatic secretion in rats with protein malnutrition. *Johns Hopkins Med. J.* **120:** 21–25, 1967.

57. Marshall, J. M., Jr. Distributions of chymotrypsinogen, procarboxyseptidase, desoxyribonuclease and ribonuclease in bovine pancreas. *Exp. Cell. Res.* **6:** 240–242, 1954.

58. Montsko, T., L. Komaromy, A. Tigyi, and K. Lissak. Cytological effect of the gastropancreatic reflex on the acinar cells of the pancreas in rana esculenta. *Acta Physiol. Acad. Sci. Hung.* **31:** 217–224, 1967.

59. Morisset, J., and J. Dunnigan. Exocrine pancreas adaptation to diet in vagotomized rats. *Rev. Canad. Biol.* **26:** 11–16, 1967.

60. Mutt, V., and J. E. Jorpes. Contemporary developments in the biochemistry of the gastrointestinal hormones. *Recent Progr. Hormone Res.* **23:** 483–503, 1967.
61. Mutt, V., and J. E. Jorpes. Isolation of aspartyl–phenylalanine amide from cholecystokinin–pancreozymin. *Biochem. Biophys. Res. Commun.* **26:** 392–397, 1967.
62. Nardi, G. L., J. M. Greep, D. A. Chambers, C. McCrae, and D. B. Skinner. Physiologic peregrinations in pancreatic perfusion. *Ann. Surg.* **158:** 830–839, 1963.
63. Pak, B. H., S. S. Hong, H. K. Pak, and S. K. Hong. Effects of acetazolamide and acid-base changes on biliary and pancreatic secretion. *Am. J. Physiol.* **210:** 624–628, 1966.
64. Palade, G. E., P. Siekevitz, and L. G. Caro. Structure, chemistry and function of the pancreatic exocrine cell. In: *The Exocrine Pancreas.* Edited by A. V. S. de Reuck and M. P. Cameron. Boston: Little, Brown & Co. 1962, pp. 23–55.
65. Peakall, D. B. Incorporation of C^{14}–orotic acid and C^{14}–amino acid into pigeon pancreas slices following cholinergic stimulation. *Proc. Soc. Exp. Biol. Med.* **126:** 198–201, 1967.
66. Perrier, C. V., D. A. Dreiling, and H. D. Janowitz. A stop-flow analysis of pancreatic secretion: The effect of transient occlusion on the electrolyte composition of pancreatic juice. *Gastroenterology* **46:** 700–705, 1964.
67. Preshaw, R. M., A. R. Cooke, and M. I. Grossman. Pancreatic secretion induced by stimulation of the pyloric gland area of the stomach. *Science* **148:** 1347–1348, 1965.
68. Preshaw, R. M. Gastric phase of pancreatic secretion. *Fed. Proc.* **25:** 1454–1457, 1966.
69. Preshaw, R. M., A. R. Cooke, and M. I. Grossman. Sham feeding and pancreatic secretion in the dog. *Gastroenterology* **50:** 171–178, 1966.
70. Preshaw, R. M., A. R. Cooke, and M. I. Grossman. Quantitative aspects of response of canine pancreas to duodenal acidification. *Am. J. Physiol.* **210:** 629–634, 1966.
71. Preshaw, R. M. Integration of nervous and hormonal mechanisms for external pancreatic secretion. In: *Handbook of Physiology.* Section 6: Alimentary Tract. Vol. II: Secretion. Edited by C. F. Code. Washington D.C.: American Physiological Society, 1967, pp. 997–1005.
72. Rawls, J. A., P. J. Wistrand, and T. H. Maren. Effects of acid–base changes and carbonic anhydrase inhibition on pancreatic secretion. *Am. J. Physiol.* **205:** 651–657, 1963.
73. Reber, H. A. and C. J. Wolf. Micropuncture study of pancreatic electrolyte secretion. *Am. J. Physiol.* **215:** 34–40, 1968.
74. Rebound, J. P., L. Pasero, and P. Desnuelle. On chymotrypsinogen and trypsinogen biosynthesis by pancreas of rats fed on a starch-rich or a casein-rich diet. *Biochem. Biophys. Res. Commun.* **17:** 347–351, 1964.
75. Rothman, S. S., and F. P. Brooks. Electrolyte secretion from the rabbit pancreas in vitro. *Am. J. Physiol.* **208:** 1171–1176, 1965.
76. Rothman, S. S., and F. P. Brooks. Pancreatic secretion in vitro in "Cl free", CO_2 free and low sodium environment. *Am. J. Physiol.* **209:** 790–796, 1965.
77. Rothman, S. S. "Non–parallel transport" of enzyme protein by the pancreas. *Nature* **213:** 460–462, 1967.

78. Rothman, S. S., and H. Wells. Enhancement of pancreatic enzyme synthesis by pancreozymin. *Am. J. Physiol.* **213:** 215–218, 1967.

79. Rune, S. J., and F. W. Henriksen. Secretory rate of gastric acid pancreatic bicarbonate in the dog after feeding. *Gastroenterology* **52:** 930–939, 1967.

80. Salman, A. J., G. Dal Borgo, M. H. Pubols, and J. McGinnis. Changes in pancreatic enzymes as a function of diet in the chick. *Proc. Soc. Exp. Biol. Med.* **126:** 694–698, 1968.

81. Sarles, H. C. Figarella, G. Prezelin, and C. Souville. Comportement different de la lipase, de l'amylase et des enzymes proteolytiques pancreatiques apres differents modes d'excitation du pancreas humain. *Bull. Soc. Chim. Biol. (Paris)* **48:** 951–957, 1966.

82. Sarles, H., R. Dani, G. Prezelin, C. Souville, and C. Figarella. Cephalic phase of pancreatic secretion in man. *Gut* **9:** 214–221, 1968.

83. Saxsena, H. C., L. S. Jensen, J. McGinnis, and J. K. Lauber. Histophysiological studies on chick pancreas as influenced by feeding raw soybean meal. *Proc. Soc. Exp. Biol. Med.* **112:** 390–393, 1963.

84. Schapiro, H., L. D. Wruble, J. W. Estes, R. Sherman, and L. G. Britt. Anticholinergic drug action on pancreatic exocrine outflow in man and dog. *Am. J. Dig. Dis.* **13:** 608–614, 1968.

85. Sesso, A. V. Valeri, and L. C. U. Junqueira. Action of thyroxine and cortisone on the secretory activity of the pancreatic acinar cell of the hypophysectomized rat. *Arch. Ges. Physiol.* **277:** 473–490, 1963.

86. Shapiro, S. H., and S. S. Lazarus. Membrane discontinuities and secretory granule formation in rabbit pancreatic acinar cells. *Exp. Molec. Path.* **6:** 320–334, 1967.

87. Siekevitz, P., and G. E. Palade. Distribution of newly synthesized amylase in microsomal subfractions of guinea pig pancreas. *J. Cell. Biol.* **30:** 519–530, 1966.

88. Sjostrand, F. S. The fine structure of the exocrine pancreas cells. In: *The Exocrine Pancreas.* Edited by A. V. S. de Reuck and M. P. Cameron. Boston: Little, Brown & Co., 1962, pp. 1–22.

89. Slayback, J. B., E. M. Swena, J. E. Thomas, and L. L. Smith. The pancreatic secretory response to topical anesthetic block of the small bowel. *Surgery* **61:** 591–595, 1967.

90. Takeda, Y., I. Suzuka, and A. Kaji. Comparative studies on specific and nonspecific binding of transfer RNA to ribosomes. *J. Biol. Chem.* **243:** 1075–1081, 1968.

91. Thomas, J. E. Neural regulation of pancreatic secretion. In: *Handbook of Physiology.* Section 6: Alimentary Tract. Vol. II: Secretion. Edited by C. F. Code. Washington, D.C.: American Physiological Society, 1967, pp. 955–968.

92. Tiscornia, O. M., and D. A. Dreiling. Does the pancreatic gland regenerate? *Gastroenterology* **51:** 267–271, 1966.

93. Van Goidsenhoven, G. E., A. F. Denk, B. A. Pfleger, and W. A. Knight. Pancreatic metabolism of Se[75] selenomethionine in dogs. *Gastroenterology* **53:** 403–411, 1967.

94. Wang, C. C., and M. I. Grossman. Physiological determination of the release of secretin and pancreozymin from intestine of dogs with transplanted pancreas. *Am. J. Physiol.* **164:** 527–545, 1951.

95. Warshawsky, H., C. P. Leblond, and B. Droz. Synthesis and migration of proteins

in the cells of the exocrine pancreas as revealed by specific activity determination from radioautographs. *J. Cell. Biol.* **16:** 1–27, 1963.

96. Wastell, C., J. Rudick, and D. A. Dreiling. Diffusion of bicarbonate across pancreatic duct epithelium. *Surg. Forum* **17:** 339–341, 1966.

97. White, T. T., G. Lundh, and D. F. Magee. Evidence for the existence of a gastropancreatic reflex. *Am. J. Physiol.* **198:** 725–728, 1960.

98. Webster, P. D., and M. P. Tyor. Effect of fasting and feeding on lipid metabolism of pigeon pancreas. *Am. J. Physiol.* **210:** 1076–1079, 1966.

99. Webster, P. D., and M. P. Tyor. Effects of intravenous pancreozymin on amino acid incorporation in vitro by pancreatic tissue. *Am. J. Physiol.* **211:** 157–160, 1966.

100. Webster, P. D., L. D. Gunn, and M. P. Tyor. Effect of in vivo pancreozymin and methacholine on pancreatic lipid metabolism. *Am. J. Physiol.* **211:** 781–785, 1966.

101. Webster, P. D., and M. P. Tyor. Effects of fasting and feeding on uridine-^{3}H incorporation into RNA by pancreas slices. *Am. J. Physiol.* **212:** 203–206, 1967.

102. Webster, P. D. III. Early effect of methacholine on pancreatic RNA synthesis. *Am. J. Physiol.* **214:** 851–855, 1968.

103. Wormsley, K. G. Response to secretin in man. *Gastroenterology* **54:** 197–209, 1968.

104. Wormsley, K. G. The action of secretin on the secretion of enzymes by the human pancreas. *Scand. J. Gastroent.* **3:** 183–188, 1968.

105. Yasuda, K., and A. H. Coons. Localization by immunofluorescence of amylase, trypsinogen and chymotrypsinogen in the acinar cells of the pig pancreas. *J. Histochem. Cytochem.* **14:** 303–313, 1968.

106. Zimmerman, M. J., D. A. Dreiling, I. R. Rosenberg, and H. D. Janowitz. Secretion of calcium by the canine pancreas. *Gastroenterology* **52:** 865–870, 1967.

Additional Reading

The Exocrine Pancreas, edited by A. V. S. de Reuck and M. P. Cameron, Boston: Little Brown & Co., 1962.

Gregory, R. A. *Secretory Mechanisms of the Gastro-intestinal Tract.* London: Edward Arnold, 1962.

Thomas, J. E. The external secretion of the Pancreas. Springfield, Ill.: Charles C Thomas, 1950.

Secretion of Bile

THE SECRETION OF BILE BY THE LIVER is probably the least studied of the gastrointestinal secretory functions. This results from the difficulties in obtaining pure bile, the presence in some species of a gallbladder which modifies the secretion before it enters the intestinal lumen, and the technical difficulties in measuring some of the constituents of bile, such as the bile acids. On the other hand, bile salts are recognized to be of great importance in the digestion and absorption of fat and are probably involved in certain disease states in man. Gallstones remain one of the more common diseases of the digestive tract, and recent studies suggest that alterations in the composition of bile may be very important in their formation.

Structural Basis of Bile Secretion

The hepatic parenchymal cell is bordered on one side by the portal venous sinusoid and on the other by the bile canaliculus. The canaliculi or bile capillaries are set off from the rest of the cell surface by condensations comparable to the terminal bars of intestinal epithelial cells (78). The secretion of bile involves the passage of substances from the blood in the sinusoids into the parenchymal cell. There, they may be stored or modified. Finally the constituents of bile are secreted into the bile canaliculus. Electron microscopy shows that the canaliculi are lined with microvilli similar to those in other secretory cells. Figure 6-1 shows a diagrammatic representation of a liver cell.

There is disagreement over the termination of the canaliculi. Some anato-

79

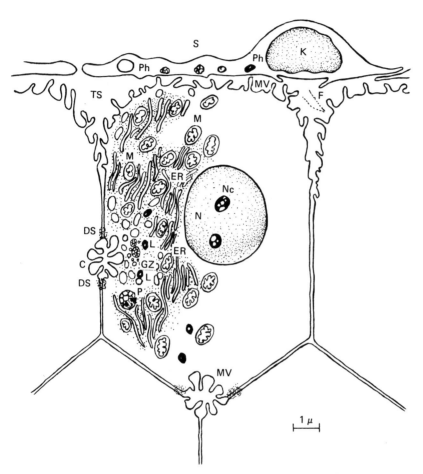

FIGURE 6-1.   Diagram of details of parenchymal liver cell seen electromicroscopically magnified about 10,000 ×. Nucleolus (Nc); nucleus (N); endoplasmic reticulum (ER); mitochondria (M); pinocytotic vacuole (V); lysome (L); Golgi zone (GZ); desmosome (DS); pigment (P); bile canaliculis (C); microvilli in canaliculi and on sinusiodal border (MV); fibers in tissue space (F); and sinusoid (S). (From H. P. Popper and F. Schaffner, (eds.). *Progress in Liver Diseases*, vol. I. New York: Grune & Stratton, 1961.)

mists believe they end blindly except for their connection to ductules. Elias cites evidence in man that they may also communicate with a space lying between the sinusoids and the hepatic parenchymal cells—the space of Disse (*21*).

The next division of the biliary tree, proceeding toward the common bile duct, is that of the ductules or cholangioles or "canals of Hering." These in turn empty into intralobular ductules. The cells lining the biliary ductules are squamous epithelial cells in the cholangioles, becoming cuboidal epithelium in the intralobular ducts and finally columnar epithelium in the main ducts.

Microvilli have been described in the duct system (21), suggesting a transport function.

Considering the liver as a whole, bile duct cells constitute 2 per cent and hepatic parenchymal cells 61 per cent of liver cells in the rat (17). There are a number of features of the ductal cells that suggest that they may play a role in bile formation. Ligation of the bile ducts leads to hypertrophy of the cholangioles (1). There is an elaborate vascular plexus about the bile ducts, reminiscent of the blood supply to the ducts of the salivary glands (45).

The extrahepatic biliary passages contain mucous glands which resemble those elsewhere in the digestive tract.

Growth and Adaptation

Little is known of the changes in the composition of bile with growth and development. Regeneration of liver cells following removal of large amounts of liver mass is a classical problem in hepatology. Humoral factors have been postulated, and recently it has been approached as a problem in the control of protein synthesis but without reference to its effect on bile secretion. It is known that the composition of the diet can affect the composition of bile. Whipple and his associates showed that high-protein diets increased the output of bile salts in bile (66). They also showed that glucose in the intestine increased the output of bilirubin (77). So the liver, like the salivary glands and pancreas, seems to be able to modify the secretion of organic molecules in reponse to changes in diet.

Relationship of Biliary Capacity to Bile Flow

As with other secretory glands, formation of secretion by gland cells must be distinguished from extrusion of secretion already resting within the ducts. The biliary tree exhibits a considerable variation in capacity, depending upon the resistance to bile flow at the entrance into the intestine (4). Figure 6-2 shows the relationship between the capacity of the biliary tree and intrabiliary pressure in the rat. This accounts for the high flow of bile following cannulation of the bile duct in cholecystectomized preparations and the much slower rate thereafter.

Composition of Bile

Hepatic bile is a viscid liquid composed primarily of water, electrolytes, bile salts, and bilirubin. It also contains cholesterol, phospholipids, proteins, and glycoproteins. In man the composition of bile is modified by the gall-

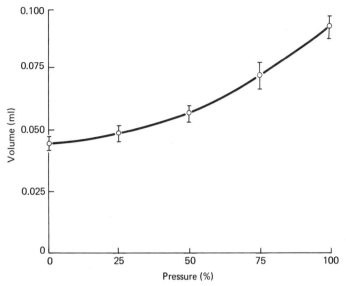

FIGURE 6-2. The relationship of the volume of bile present in the biliary tree to intrabiliary pressure (expressed as a percentage of the mean maximum pressure attained). The mean and the standard error of the mean for twelve animals are shown. (From G. Barber-Riley. Measurement of the capacity of the biliary tree. In: *The Biliary System.* Edited by W. I. Taylor. Oxford: Blackwell Scientific Publications, 1965.)

bladder, as will be discussed under absorption. Table 6-1 shows the composition of human hepatic bile as determined in two studies (*13,71*). It should be recalled that some of the data were collected from T tubes following exploration of the common duct and that even that from individuals without biliary tract disease was obtained under anesthesia at laparotomy (*13*). It can be seen that the concentrations of sodium, potassium, and chloride do not differ greatly

TABLE 6-1
Composition of Human Hepatic Bile

Sodium	146–165 mEq/L(71)
Potassium	2.7–4.9
Calcium	2.5–4.8
Magnesium	1.4–3.0
Chloride	88–115
Bicarbonate	27– 55
Bile salts	40–160
Calcium	21 mg/100 ml
Bile salts	1,800
Cholesterol	130
Bilirubin	92
Lecithin	710

from those in plasma, while the concentrations of bicarbonate and calcium are significantly greater. In dogs the composition of bile changes promptly upon interruption of the enterohepatic circulation, with a marked fall in the concentration of bile salts.

Proteins are present in bile in low concentrations—20 mg/100 ml in human bile according to Burnett (13). Albumin can be identified and free amino acids have been reported. (57). Cholesterol is present in concentrations similar to serum (52). The solubility of cholesterol in bile is related to the concentrations of bile salts and phospholipids. The principal phospholipid in bile is lecithin, with small amounts of cephalin, sphingomyelin, and lysolecithin (5). Lecithin itself consists of seven different fractions on silica gel electrophoresis (48).

Bouchier and Cooperband found a macromolecular aggregate associated with bilirubin in human hepatic bile with a molecular weight of 11,000 to 20,000. They found it associated with cholesterol, phospholipids, and bile salts, and considered it to represent a micellar aggregate (11).

The pH of hepatic bile is usually near 7, and it is isosmotic with respect to plasma. The bile salts are primarily conjugates of cholic acid, with taurine or glycine in varying percentages in different species. In man the ratio of taurocholic to glycocholic acid is about 2 to 1. Interruption of the enterohepatic circulation in the rabbit results in a change of the principal bile acid from glycodeoxycholic acid to glycocholic acid (26).

Mechanisms of Bile Formation

The most significant theory for the formation of bile in modern times has been the concept of Sperber that certain organic anions, particularly bile salts, move from the hepatic parenchymal cell into the canaliculus by an active transport process. Water and electrolyte follow in response to an osmotic gradient. There is little restriction to the passage of sodium, chloride, and potassium between bile and plasma (67). Dvorak and Horky noted changes in the ultrastructure of hepatic cells during alterations in secretory rate and found that the most active structures were the Golgi complex and mitochondria (20). There were no changes in the endoplasmic reticulum, ribosomes, or cell inclusions.

In dogs under anesthesia, a maximum rate of taurocholate secretion in bile of about 9 μmoles/kg/min was achieved, with synthetic intravenous taurocholate given at about 12 μmoles/kg/min. I have seen hemolysis and hematuria in conscious dogs at taurocholate infusion rates of about 8 μmoles/kg/min. Bile flow at this maximal secretory rate was about 1.4 ml/15 min (54a). The same investigators found that the extraction rate of synthetic taurocholate infused at the rate of 2.9 μmoles/kg/min was 92 per cent (55).

Okishio and Nair (53) found that more than 50 per cent of bile acids except deoxycholic acid was located in the cytoplasmic compartment of hepatic cells. Twice as much deoxycholic acid was present in microsomes as in the nuclear and mitochondrial fractions, and a much larger proportion was present in these organelles than in the cytoplasmic compartment. The other bile acids were divided equally among the particulate elements. Enzymes involved in hydroxylation were located in microsomes and mitochondria.

In man and most mammals, the two main primary bile acids are cholic (trihydroxy acid) and chenodeoxycholic acid (dihydroxy acid). The half-life of cholic acid in man was found to be about 3 days, and the production of total bile acids about 500 to 700 mg/day (8). About 300 mg was excreted in the feces daily.

Bilirubin contributes relatively little to the osmotic activity of bile, yet it enters bile in much greater concentration than that in serum. A chemically related dye, the sodium salt of fluorescein (uranin), can be followed under the microscope from the blood to the bile (27). It appears in the sinusoids a few seconds after intravenous injection and a minute later in the bile capillaries. It can be seen distributed throughout the liver cell and gradually leaving through the bile capillaries.

In order to be secreted into the bile, bilirubin must be conjugated with glucoronide or to a lesser degree sulfate. The former step occurs in the parenchymal cell in the presence of the enzyme, or enzymes, glucuronyl transferase (2). Lester and Klein found that 90 per cent of the bilirubin and mesobilirubin was secreted as glucuronide, but a major fraction of mesobilirubinogen and i-urobilin appeared intact and unaltered (43).

The secretion of bilirubin is to a degree independent of bile flow. In mice and rats, bile flow was more sensitive to changes in temperature than the secretion of bilirubin (60).

The lecithins of bile are formed in the liver, probably derived from separate pools (3). The incorporation of plasma free fatty acids into bile lipids has been studied in two human subjects (62). Plasma and bile lipids rose in parallel after ^{14}C-labeled palmitate, reaching maximal activity in two hours. The label was recovered in biliary lecithin, indicating a small phospholipid pool in the liver prior to secretion.

The mechanisms by which a number of synthetic or foreign substances enter bile has given insight into the formation of bile. Sulfobromophthalein (BSP) is a dye with a purple color in alkaline solution which is chemically related to bilirubin and can be demonstrated to enter a storage phase within the hepatic parenchymal cells before it is secreted into the bile. It can be shown to compete with bile acids in a common secretory mechanism (54b). The passage of a series of ferrioxamines into the bile in perfused rat livers was related to their liposolubility. With increasing solubility, biliary excretion increased and active transport became a more dominant feature (46). Ouabain (42) and chlorothiazide (30) are actively transported into bile by mechanisms involving carriers distinct from other naturally occurring anions.

Cellular Metabolism and Bile Secretion

As with other digestive secretory glands, metabolic inhibitors may be used to detect the role of various energy-releasing pathways in bile formation. In anesthetized dogs, acetazolamide and p-chloromercuribenzoic acid had no significant effect on bile flow. Phloridzin inhibited the output of bile pigment without affecting flow, while dinitrophenol increased bile flow (68). It will be necessary to measure the composition of bile in such experiments to determine more specifically the site of action of the inhibitors.

In the perfused rat liver, acetazolamide was also without effect, but cyanide reduced bile secretion (10). Again phloridzin inhibited bilirubin transport but increased bile flow.

Control of Bile Secretion

Under normal circumstances the secretion of bile is thought to be controlled by the level of bile salts in the portal venous blood (8). Interruption of the enterohepatic circulation by diverting bile to the outside increased the hepatic synthesis of bile salts to more than ten times the normal rate in rats (7). In dogs, however, Neistadt et al. found no alteration in resting bile flow after acute or chronic portacaval shunts (51).

Kelly and Klopper found that the pO_2 of bile was closer to that in arterial than portal blood. Hyperbaric oxygen increased the pO_2 of both bile and arterial blood but not portal venous blood (39). Hypertonic solutions given intravenously reduce bile flow as they do other secretions (14). Alkalosis increases the response of bile flow to secretin, while acidosis reduces it (56).

Much of present speculation about the control of bile flow is based upon a division of bile into components, each subject to specific controlling factors. Wheeler and Ramos found that secretin stimulated bile secretion characterized by high bicarbonate concentrations and suggested that a two-component theory similar to that for the stomach might account for the observations. One component was related to the active transport of bile salts while the other was a bicarbonate-rich fluid similar to pancreatic juice (74). Later Wheeler and his colleagues produced indirect evidence that the bicarbonate-rich fluid was added in the ducts rather than in the canaliculus (75).

Since then a variety of techniques have pointed to a role of the ducts in bile secretion. On the basis of stop-flow studies in rabbits, Chenderovitch postulated a proximal segment where bile salts were secreted and reabsorption of water and electrolyte occurred. In the distal segment, a fluid with a composition similar to that of primary bile with respect to sodium and chloride might be added. Goblet cells might account for the addition of potassium (15). Ross and Silen found increases in bicarbonate concentrations in bile from the ducts in stop-flow experiments in dogs (61). Forker used Diodrast transit times and the clearance of mannitol and erythritol in guinea pigs to support the concept of two sites of bile formation (23,24).

London and his associates measured a negative mucosal to serosal potential difference across the bile duct in guinea pigs and dogs. They concluded that there was an active bicarbonate transport mechanism in the ducts and that sodium chloride might be reabsorbed by a neutral coupled mechanism (44).

More recently, Wheeler et al. have suggested a fourth mechanism— canalicular secretion at the rate of 0.1 ml/min in dogs under the influence of anticholinergic drugs, which is independent of the secretion of bile salts (76).

Structural changes in the ducts coincident with cholestasis are consistent with a role of the ducts in bile formation (66).

HORMONAL CONTROL

The major gastrointestinal hormones—secretin, gastrin, and pancreozymin-cholecystokinin—have already been discussed. The first two have definite effects on bile secretion and the third probably does. The problem now becomes that of determining their physiologic significance. Synthetic secretin has been shown to produce a choleresis in dogs, disposing of the old claim that the choleretic action of secretin was due to a contaminant (72). The bicarbonate concentration of bile stimulated by secretin was found to be as great as 60 mEq/L (74) and calculated in bile from a perfused pig liver as 124 mEq/L (28,29). O'Maille et al. found that maximal BSP secretory rate was unchanged by secretin, indicating no common mechanism (54b). In man, Waitman et al. found that secretin increased bile flow from T tubes with an increase in bicarbonate concentration and a fall in chloride (73). Acetazolamide reduced the rise in bicarbonate with secretin. Scratcherd found a similar response in cats, with bicarbonate concentrations reaching 40 mEq/L (64). However, secretin had no effect on the flow of bile in the rabbit. The response to secretin reaches a maximum, and it was possible that the rabbit was already secreting at this rate.

There remains the problem of physiologic significance. Jorpes et al. doubt a significant role of secretin, since the dose must be relatively high in relation to that required for pancreatic secretion to be effective (36). They suggested that pancreozymin-cholecystokinin might be more effective. However, later reports from the same investigators question the role of the hormone in mediation of the feeding response (35). Results with the synthetic hormone should clarify the matter.

In 1965, Jones et al. reported that irrigation of an antral pouch with peptone or liver extract but not saline caused a choleresis (33). Later Zaterka and Grossman found that pure gastrin caused a choleresis in gastrectomized dogs (79). Finally Nahrwold et al. showed that irrigation of an antral pouch with acetylcholine in neutral solution caused a choleresis but not if the solution had a low pH (50). There still remains the question of physiologic significance.

Glucagon also causes a choleresis in dog (22) and man (69). Morris and his associates found that the choleresis after glucagon differed from that after secretin (47). There was a transient increased output of bile salts and an increase in hepatic blood flow.

Catecholamines alter the flow and composition of bile in anesthetized dogs. Norepinephrine reduced bile flow, epinephrine had little effect, and isoprenaline had a biphasic effect (38). Isoprenaline also increased the concentration of bile salts, decreased that of cholesterol, and had no effect on bilirubin concentration.

Other hormonal effects on bile secretion seem to fall into the category of permissive actions. Hypophysectomy reduced the secretin of conjugated bilirubin in rats (25), and hypopituitarism in man was associated with a 43 per cent decrease in the maximal secretory rate of BSP without change in the storage factor (63). Beher et al. found that the rate of bile acid elimination was the rate-limiting step in the secretion of bile acids after hypophysectomy in rats (6).

Thorbjarnarson and Pitman found that the concentration of phospholipids rose in both the plasma and bile in patients with hypothyroidism. There was no correlation between the bile and serum cholesterol (70).

NERVOUS CONTROL

Fritz and Brooks found that insulin hypoglycemia led to a choleresis independently of its effect on gastric secretion. The effect was blocked by vagotomy or anticholinergic drugs (22). Preisig et al. claimed that an infusion of anticholinergic drug reduced the variability of bile flow in the conscious dog (59). The observation that the choleresis after feeding was abolished by vagotomy suggested that neural control had physiologic significance (22). However, the role of vagal release of gastrin under normal circumstances is unclear. Antrectomy nearly abolished the choleresis after insulin, but left the feeding response unchanged. Sham feeding had little effect on bile flow despite the usual gastric response (58,40). Another vagal stimulant, 2-deoxy-D-glucose, is much less effective as a choleretic than insulin although equivalent in its action on acid secretion (41). It is interesting that insulin is present in bile (16).

Posterior hypothalamic electrical stimulation increased bile flow in acute experiments in cats (9).

BLOOD FLOW AND BILE SECRETION

Pressures in the biliary tree usually exceed that in the portal vein by 50 per cent, thereby ruling out filtration as a mechanism in bile secretion as in the salivary glands (12). Over a wide range of perfusion rates in the isolated rat liver, bile flow remained constant. In anesthetized dogs, bile secretion was independent of hepatic arterial pressure but increased by 60 per cent after periarterial neuronectomy (80).

OTHER CONTROLLING FACTORS

The choleresis after feeding in the presence of an interrupted enterohepatic circulation was characterized by an increased output of water and electrolyte. When bile was returned to the intestine, bile flow and the output of bile salts increased (50). Muscular work increased the output of bile salt and cholesterol in rats (19). In man with a T tube, elevation of the side arm of the tube results in an increased concentration of bile acids and the serum cholesterol (18).

SUMMARY

The secretion of bile by the liver is under the control of the enterohepatic circulation of bile salts. Cholinergic influences and the vagus exert a controlling influence on the nonbile-salt component. Diet can also modify secretion. The physiologic control exercised by gastrin, secretin, and pancreozymin remains to be determined.

Bile Secretion in Man

There is little information on the control of hepatic bile secretion in normal man. In patients with T tubes, secretin and glucagon exert choleretic effects similar to those in experimental animals.

Pathophysiology

The accumulation of bilirubin in the blood (jaundice) may be due to failure of uptake of bilirubin from its albumin-bilirubin complex in the sinusoids (Gilbert's disease), failure of conjugation due to a lack of glucuronyl transferase, or failure of the secretory mechanism (Dubin-Johnson syndrome), as well as dysfunction of the parenchymal cells (hepatitis or cirrhosis), mechanical obstruction of the common bile duct (common duct stone, pancreatic cancer), or hemolysis (spherocytosis). Inability of the liver to synthesize bile salts may lead to malabsorption of fat due to maldigestion as a result of failure to form micelles. Prolonged drainage of bile may cause loss of bone substance due to malabsorption of calcium. Recent evidence implicates the formation of lithocholic acid in the production of intrahepatic obstruction (cholestasis) (32).

References

1. Andrews, W. H. H. Bile duct cells and bile secretion. In: *Liver Function*. Edited by R. W. Brauer. Washington, D.C.: A.I.B.S., 1958. pp. 241–248.
2. Arias, I. The excretion of conjugated bilirubin by the liver cell. *Medicine* **45:** 513–515, 1966.
3. Balint, J. A., D. A. Beeler, D. H. Treble, and H. L. Spitzer. Studies in the biosynthesis of hepatic and biliary lecithins. *J. Lipid Res.* **8:** 486–493, 1967.
4. Barber-Riley, G. Measurement of the capacity of the biliary tree. In: *The Biliary System*. Edited by W. Taylor. Oxford: Blackwell Scientific Publications, 1965, pp. 89–97.
5. Barton, P. G., and J. Glover. The role of the biliary phospholipids in dispersing sterols prior to the absorption from the intestine. In: *The Biliary System*. Edited by W. Taylor. Oxford: Blackwell Scientific Publications, 1965, pp. 189–198.
6. Beher, W. T., B. Rao, M. E. Beher, and J. Bertasius. Bile acid synthesis in normal and hypophysectomized rats; a rate study using cholestyramine. *Proc. Soc. Exp. Biol. Med.* **124:** 1193–1197, 1967.
7. Bergstrom, S. Bile acid formation and secretion. In: *Liver Function*. Edited by R. A. Brauer. Washington D.C.: A.I.B.S., 1958. pp. 310–324.
8. Bergstrom, S., and H. Danielsson. Formation and metabolism of bile acids. In: *The Biliary System*. Edited by W. Taylor, Oxford: Blackwell Scientific Publications, 1965, pp. 117–128.
9. Birnbaum, D., and S. Feldman. Effect of hypothalamic stimulation on bile secretion. *J. Lab. Clin. Med.* **60:** 914–922, 1962.
10. Bizard, G. Enzyme inhibitors and biliary secretion. In: *The Biliary System*. Edited by W. Taylor, Oxford: Blackwell Scientific Publications, 1965, pp. 315–324.
11. Bouchier, I. A. D., and S. R. Cooperband. Isolation and characterization of a macromolecular aggregate associated with bilirubin. *Clin. Chim. Acta.* **15:** 291–302, 1967.
12. Brauer, R. W. Hepatic blood supply and the secretion of bile. In: *The Biliary System*. Edited by W. Taylor, Oxford: Blackwell Scientific Publications, 1965, pp. 41–67.
13. Burnett, W. The pathogenesis of gall stones. In: *The Biliary System*. Edited by W. Taylor, Oxford: Blackwell Scientific Publications, 1965, pp. 601–618.
14. Chenderovitch, J., E. Phocas, and M. Rautureau. Effects of hypertonic solutions on bile formation. *Am. J. Physiol.* **205:** 863–867, 1963.
15. Chenderovitch, J. Stop-flow analysis of bile secretion. *Am. J. Physiol.* **214:** 86–93, 1968.
16. Daniel, P. M., and J. R. Henderson. Insulin in bile and other body fluids. *Lancet* **1:** 1256–1257, 1967.
17. Daoust, R. The cell population of liver tissue and the cytological reference bases. In: *Liver Function*. Edited by R. W. Brauer. Washington, D.C.: A.I.B.S., 1958, pp. 3–10.
18. DePalma, R. G., S. Levey, P. H. Hartman, and C. A. Hubay. Bile acids and serum cholesterol following T-tube drainage. *Arch. Surg.* **94:** 271–276, 1967.
19. Duperray, D., and H. Pacheco. Influence du travail musculaire sur de debit et

la composition de la bile chez le rat. *C. R. Acad. Sci.* **263:** Ser.D. 1887–1890, 1966.

20. Dvorak, M., and D. Horky. Submikroskopische Struktur der Leberzelle nach Beeinflussung ihrer Sekretiostatigkeit. *Z. Zellforsch.* **76:** 486–497, 1967.

21. Elias, H. Embryology, histology and anatomy of the biliary system. In: *The Biliary System.* Edited by W. Taylor. Oxford: Blackwell Scientific Publications, 1965, pp. 1–13.

22. Fritz, M. E., and F. P. Brooks. Control of bile flow in the conscious dog. *Am. J. Physiol.* **204:** 825–828, 1963.

23. Forker, E. L. Two sites of bile formation as determined by mannitol and erythritol clearance in the guinea pig. *J. Clin. Invest.* **46:** 1189–1195, 1967.

24. Forker, E. L., and C. A. M. Hogben. Diodrast transit time in guinea pig biliary tree. *Am. J. Physiol.* **212:** 104–112, 1967.

25. Gartner, L. M., and I. M. Arias. Pituitary regulation of bilirubin excretion by the liver. *J. Clin. Invest.* **45:** 1011, 1966.

26. Gregg, J. A., and L. R. Poley. Excretion of bile acids in normal rabbits. *Am. J. Physiol.* **211:** 1147–1151, 1966.

27. Hanzon, V. Dye secretion and dye uptake by the liver. In: *Liver Function.* Edited by R. W. Rauer. Washington, D.C.: A.I.B.S., 1958, pp. 281–290.

28. Hardison, W. G., and J. C. Norman. Effect of bile salt and secretin upon bile flow from the isolated perfused pig liver. *Gastroenterology* **53:** 412–417, 1967.

29. Hardison, W. G., and J. C. Norman. Electrolyte composition of the secretin fraction of bile from the perfused pig liver. *Am. J. Physiol.* **214:** 758–763, 1968.

30. Hart, L. G., and L. S. Schanker. Active transport of chlorthiazide into bile. *Am. J. Physiol.* **211:** 643–646, 1966.

31. Hauton, J. C., R. Depieds, and H. Sarles. Proteins in Bile. In: *The Biliary System.* Edited by W. Taylor. Oxford: Blackwell Scientific Publications, 1965, pp. 433–448.

32. Javitt, N. B., and S. Emerman. Effect of sodium taurolithocholate on bile flow and bile acid excretion. *J. Clin. Invest.* **47:** 1002–1014, 1968.

33. Jones, R. S., K. C. Powell, and F. P. Brooks. The role of the gastric antrum in the control of bile flow. *Surg. Forum* **16:** 386–387, 1965.

34. Jones, R. S., and F. P. Brooks. Role of pyloric antrum in choleresis after insulin and feeding. *Am. J. Physiol.* **213:** 1406–1408, 1967.

35. Jonson, G., G. Svertengren, and L. Tulin. The effect of cholecystokinin-pancreozymin preparations on hepatic bile output in fasting and digesting dogs. *Acta Physiol. Scand.* **69:** 23–28, 1967.

36. Jorpes, E., V. Mutt, G. Jonson, L. Thulin, and L. Sundman. The influence of secretin and cholecystokinin on bile flow. In: *The Biliary System.* Edited by W. Taylor, Oxford: Blackwell Scientific Publications, 1965, pp. 293–301.

37. Kasture, A. V., and A. K. Dorle. The effect of isoprenaline on the bile secretion of anesthetized dogs. *Current Sci.* **36:** 178–179, 1967.

38. Kasture, A. V., D. S. Shingvekar, and A. K. Dorle. Effect of adrenaline, noradrenaline and isoprenaline on hepatic bile secretion of anesthetized dogs. *Nature* **212:** 1598–1599, 1966.

39. Kelly, K. A., and P. J. Klopper. Influence of isobaric and hyperbaric oxygen on biliary pO_2 and the mechanics of bile flow. *Am. J. Physiol.* **212:** 1017–1019, 1967.

40. Konstantinov, M. V. The mechanisms of bile formation and secretion. *Bull. Exp. Biol. Med. USSR* **62:** 1099–1101, 1966 (Engl. Transl.).

41. Konturek, S. J., A. Kieta-Fayda, and K. Moczurad. The influence of gastrin analogues and 2-deoxy-D-glucose on bile secretion. *Am. J. Digest. Dis.* **12:** 955–961, 1967.

42. Kupferberg, H. J., and L. S. Schanker. Biliary secretion of oubain-^{3}H and its uptake by liver slices in the rat. *Am. J. Physiol.* **214:** 1048–1053, 1968.

43. Lester, R., and P. D. Klein. Bile pigment excretion: a comparison of the biliary excretion of bilirubin and bilirubin derivatives. *J. Clin. Invest.* **45:** 1839–1846, 1966.

44. London, C. D., J. M. Diamond, and F. P. Brooks. Electrical potential differences in the biliary tree. *Biochim. Biophys. Acta* **150:** 509–517, 1968.

45. Maegraith, B. G. Bile duct cells and their blood supply. In: *Liver Function.* Edited by R. W. Brauer. Washington, D.C.: A.I.B.S., 1958, pp. 235–240.

46. Meyer-Brunot, H. G., and H. Keberle. Biliary excretion of ferrioxamines of varying liposolubility in perfused rat liver. *Am. J. Physiol.* **214:** 1193–1200, 1968.

47. Morris, T. Q., G. F. Sardi, and S. E. Bradley. Character of glucagon induced choleresis. *Fed. Proc.* **26:** 774, 1967.

48. Nakayama, F., and S. Kawamura. Composition of biliary lecichins. *Clin. Chim. Acta* **17:** 53–58, 1967.

49. Nahrwold, D. L., A. R. Cooke, and M. I. Grossman. Choleresis induced by stimulation of the gastric antrum. *Gastroenterology* **52:** 18–22, 1967.

50. Nahrwold, D. L., and M. I. Grossman. Secretion of bile in response to food with and without bile in the intestine. *Gastroenterology* **53:** 11–17, 1967.

51. Neistadt, A., J. F. C. Lima, and S. I. Schwartz. Effects of portacaval shunts on flow and composition of bile. *Surgery* **61:** 427–431, 1967.

52. Norman, A. Physico-chemical properties of bile constituents. In: *The Biliary System.* Edited by W. Taylor, Oxford: Blackwell Scientific Publications, 1965, pp. 165–174.

53. Okishio, T., and P. P. Nagir. Studies on bile acids; some observations on the intracellular localization of major bile acids in rat liver. *Biochemistry* **5:** 3662–3668, 1966.

54a. O'Maille, E. R. L., T. G. Richards, and A. H. Short. Acute Taurine depletion and maximal rates of hepatic conjugation and secretion of cholic acid in the dog. *J. Physiol. London* **180:** 67–79, 1965.

54b. O'Maille, E. R. L., T. G. Richards, and A. H. Short. Factors determining the maximal rate of organic anion secretion by the liver and further evidence on the hepatic site of action of the hormone secretion. *J. Physiol. London* **186:** 424–438, 1966.

55. O'Maille, E. R. L., T. G. Richards, and A. H. Short. The influence of conjugation of cholic acid on its uptake and secretion: Hepatic extraction of taurocholate and cholate in the dog. *J. Physiol. London* **189:** 337–350, 1967.

56. Pak, B. H., S. S. Hong, H. K. Pak, and S. K. Hong. Effects of acetazolamide and acid-base changes on biliary and pancreatic secretion. *Am. J. Physiol.* **210:** 624–628, 1966.

57. Pappo, A. La separation par la chromatographie sur papier, de plusieurs acides amines libres dans la bile hepatique humaine. *Acta Gastroenterol. Belg.* **29:** 949–954, 1966.

58. Powell, K. C., L. C. Miller, and F. P. Brooks. Effect of sham feeding on bile flow in cholecystectomized dogs. *Proc. Exp. Biol. Med.* **118:** 481–483, 1965.

59. Preisig, R., H. L. Cooper, and H. O. Wheeler. The relationship between taurocholate secretion rate and bile production in the unanesthetized dog during cholinergic blockade and during secretin administration. *J. Clin. Invest.* **41:** 1152–1162, 1962.

60. Roberts, R. J., C. D. Klaasen, and G. L. Plaa. Maximum biliary excretion of bilirubin and sulfobromophthalein during anesthesia-induced alteration of rectal temperature. *Proc. Soc. Exp. Biol. Med.* **125:** 313–316, 1967.

61. Ross, H., and W. Silen. The influence of the biliary ducts on the composition of bile. *Gastroenterology* **54:** 1265, 1968.

62. Sasaki, H. F. Schaffner, and H. Popper. Bile ductules in cholestasis: Morphologic evidence for secretion and absorption in man. *Lab Invest.* **16:** 84–95, 1967.

63. Schersten, T., A. Gottfries, S. Nilsson, and B. Samuelsson. Incorporation of plasma free fatty acids into bile lipids in man. *Life Sci.* **6:** 1775–1780, 1967.

64. Schmidt, M. L., L. M. Gartner, and I. M. Arias. Studies of hepatic excretory function. III. Effects of hypopituitarism on the hepatic excretion of sulfobromophthalein sodium in man. *Gastroenterology* **52:** 998–1002, 1967.

65. Scratcherd, T. Electrolyte composition and control of biliary secretion in the cat and rabbit. In: *The Biliary System.* Edited by W. Taylor. Oxford: Blackwell Scientific Publications. 1965, pp. 515–529.

66. Smith, H. P., and G. H. Whipple. Bile salt metabolism. II. Influence of meat and meat extractives, liver and kidney, egg yolk and yeast in the diet. *J. Biol. Chem.* **80:** 671–684, 1928.

67. Sperber, I. Biliary secretion of organic anions and its influence on bile flow. In: *The Biliary System.* Edited by W. Taylor. Oxford: Blackwell Scientific Publications, 1965, pp. 457–467.

68. Stone, S. L. Energy requirements for bile secretion. In: *The Biliary System.* Edited by W. Taylor. Oxford: Blackwell Scientific Publications, 1965, pp. 277–292.

69. Sweeting, J. G. The effect of glucagon on bile and pancreatic juice. *Gastroenterology* **54:** 1276, 1968.

70. Thorbjarnarson, B., and J. Pitman. Serum and bile lipids in altered thyroid function. *Arch. Surg.* **94:** 231–234, 1967.

71. Thureborn, E. Human hepatic bile: composition changes due to altered enterohepatic circulation. *Acta Chir. Scand.* Suppl. 303, pp. 1–63, 1962.

72. Vagne, M., F. Stening, F. Brooks, and M. I. Grossman. Physiological properties of synthetic secretin. *Gastroenterology* **54:** 1280, 1968.

73. Waitman, A. M., W. P. Dyck, and H. D. Janowitz. The effect of secretin and acetazolamide on the electrolyte secretion of the liver in man. *Gastroenterology* **54:** 1280, 1968.

74. Wheeler, H. O., and O. L. Ramos. Determinants of the flow and composition of bile in the unanesthetized dog during constant infusions of sodium taurocholate. *J. Clin. Invest.* **39:** 161–170, 1960.

75. Wheeler, H. O., and P. L. Mancusi-Ungaro. Role of bile ducts during secretin choleresis in dogs. *Am. J. Physiol.* **210:** 1153–1159, 1966.

76. Wheeler, H. O., E. D. Ross, and S. E. Bradley. Canalicular bile production in dogs. *Am. J. Physiol.* **214:** 866–874, 1968.

77. Whipple, G. H., and C. W. Hooper. Bile pigment metabolism. II. Bile pigment output influenced by diet. *Am. J. Physiol.* **40:** 349–359, 1916.

78. Wilson, J. W. Hepatic structure in relation to function. In: *Liver Function,* edited by R. W. Brauer, Washington, D.C.: A.I.B.S., 1958, pp. 175–192.

79. Zaterka, S., and M. I. Grossman. The effect of gastrin and histamine on the secretion of bile. *Gastroenterology* **50:** 500–505, 1966.

80. Zochler, C. E., H. Droge, and R. Friedel, Cholorese und Leberdurchblutung. *Z. Gastroenterol.* **4:** 204–211, 1966.

Additional Reading

Liver Function, edited by R. W. Brauer. Washington, D.C.: A.I.B.S., 1968.

The Biliary System, edited by W. Taylor. Oxford: Blackwell Scientific Publications, 1965.

Secretions of the Intestines

IN THE PAST, THE INTESTINES WERE THOUGHT to contribute secretion to the lumen of the digestive tract in much the same fashion as other secretory glands. The term *succus entericus* was a reflection of this. More recently, the constituents of the succus have been gradually eliminated with the exception of Brunner's glands. Improved techniques of collection indicated that many of the enzymatic activities previously assigned to the succus were due to intracellular enzymes in cells shed into the digestive tract as a result of the high rate of cellular renewal. In the proximal gut, the flux of water and electrolyte from lumen to blood greatly exceeded that in the opposite direction. This left only the ileum with the possibility of a secretion of bicarbonate as an active process.

Several recent developments may alter the situation. Certain diarrheal diseases such as cholera and islet-cell tumors seem to be the result of hypersecretion. Study of the small intestine in vivo consistently suggests secretion of bicarbonate in the ileum, and certain villous tumors of the colon secrete sufficient potassium to produce significant hypokalemia.

Evidence of a morphologic basis for intestinal secretion has come from studies of the ultrastructure of the intestinal mucosa. Trier suggested four types of cells with secretory functions—goblet cells, Paneth cells, enterochromaffin cells, and undifferentiated crypt cells (20). Goblet cells contain secretory granules which stain for mucopolysaccharides. Enterochromaffin cells contain serotonin (16). Secretory granules can be demonstrated in Paneth cells and undifferentiated crypt cells, but their nature is unknown.

The techniques of electron microscopy and autoradiography have added to our knowledge of goblet cells. Strong stimulation of the rat colon with mustard oil (6) led to discharge of mucous granules, but most workers believe that goblet cells secrete continuously (15). Goblet cells increase in number from midjejunum to terminal ileum (20). The apical margin contains a few microvilli, as shown in Figure 7-1. Earlier investigators considered secretion from goblet cells to be an example of apocrine secretion in which a portion of the apical cytoplasm was shed with the granules. This may be a peculiar feature of the guinea pig (8). In most situations, the granules of mucus escape from the intact cell (merocrine secretion) (17,20). In rats, the mucous granules appeared continuous with each other. There were perforations in the apical cytoplasm, and mucous granules with intact membranes could be seen in the lumen (17). The terminal web of goblet cells is poorly developed, and the discrete mucous granules measure 3 μ in diameter, enclosed in a membranous envelope (20). Some proliferation of goblet cells occurs (20).

Autoradiographic studies with labeled sulfur showed that goblet cells took up the label in differing patterns throughout the intestine (12). There were also differences between species (10).

Ultrastructural studies showed that labeled glucose appeared in the Golgi membranes of goblet cells in the colon within 5 minutes. At 20 minutes it could be identified in mucous granules. Forty minutes later the label was distributed throughout the supranuclear region, and at 4 hours it was confined to the apical cytoplasm (15). Freeman interpreted his observations as showing protein synthesis in the endoplasmic reticulum, which was then transmitted to the Golgi apparatus. There it was combined with acid mucopolysaccharide and glycoproteins synthesized by the Golgi apparatus (8). The latter process may have involved sulfation (1).

Trier and his associates demonstrated the secretion of granules from Paneth cells (21). Feeding had no effect on the synthesis or secretion of granules, but pilocarpine stimulated both. Atropine inhibited secretion but had no effect on synthesis. The chemical nature of the granules is unknown.

Enterochromaffin cells include argentaffin and argyrophil cells. The presence of these cells can be correlated with serotonin, as noted in the chapter on gastric secretion (16). In man, serotonin is present in highest amounts in the duodenum and decreases caudally. The same is true of enterochromaffin cells. The physiologic significance of serotonin is unknown.

The undifferentiated crypt cells also contain secretory granules which stain for mucopolysaccharides. The granules as well as portions of the apical cytoplasm (apocrine secretion) have been seen in the lumen in man (20).

Finally, the use of immunofluorescence for staining cells has identified immunoglobulins in intestinal epithelium. Primarily seen in plasma cells, immunoglobulin A (IgA) predominated throughout the intestinal tract in man in contrast to the plasma, where IgG is the principal component (4). Interestingly, this was also true of the rectal secretion of two patients with villous tumors (13).

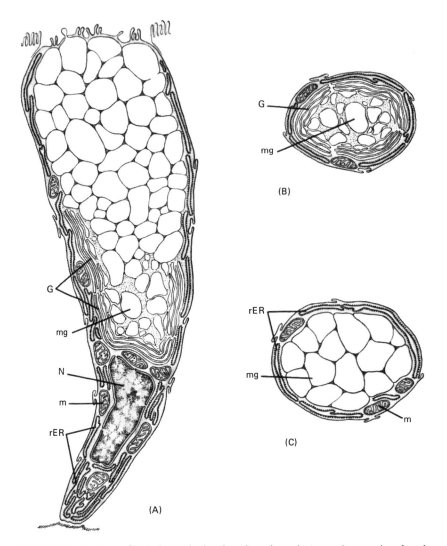

FIGURE 7-1.   Semischematic drawings based on electron micrographs of surface goblet cells of colon of 10-gm rats. A: In longitudinal section, the Golgi complex (G) forms a U above the nucleus (N). It is composed of several stacks of saccules. Each stack includes 7 to 12 saccules (only 4 of which are depicted here). There seem to be transitions between the most central saccules and the loosely packed mucigen granules (mg) which occupy the central portion of the supranuclear area. Above, closely packed mucigen granules occupy the cell apex (m, mitochondria; rER, roughed-surfaced endoplasmic reticulum or ergastoplasm). B: Transverse section through the supranuclear region. The Golgi complex (G) forms a ring around mucigen granules (mg). The Golgi complex in turn is rimmed by a narrow margin of cytoplasm. C: Transverse section above the Golgi complex. The group of apical mucigen granules (mg) is rimmed by cytoplasm. Rough endoplasmic reticulum (rER) and mitochondria (m) may be distinguished. (From C. P. Leblond. *J. Cell Biol.* **30:** 122, 1966.)

Physiologic studies have usually concerned themselves with the secretion of Brunner's glands or the glands in the remainder of the small intestine. In man, Brunner's glands extend from the pylorus to the minor pancreatic duct. They can be identified in clusters as far down as the jejunum in about a third of subjects (9). The acini and tubules are lined with a single type of cell. In dogs electrolyte composition of secretion from pouches lined with Brunner's glands was Sodium 145 mEq/L, chloride 136, potassium 6.3, and bicarbonate 17 (2,3). The secretion was very viscid, with a pH of 8.2 to 9.3 (9). It contained peptic activity and a mucinase. The control of secretion from Brunner's glands is poorly understood. Crude tissue extracts, but not secretin or gastrin, stimulate secretion. Motility per se had no exciting effect (2). Urecholine stimulated motility but not secretion (3). Denervation had no effect on spontaneous secretion (22).

Pouches of the entire duodenum in dogs secreted about 300 ml/day, presumably in a greater part from the crypts of Lieberkuhn (11). Amylase, lipase, saccharase, and lactase activity was present. However, Florey and his colleagues could detect only enterokinase and amylase activity when cellular debris was excluded (22). Insulin hypoglycemia had no effect on whole duodenum pouches (11). Small bowel deoxyribonucleic acid content collected from the lumen correlates with intestinal epithelial turnover (5).

Other evidence of the role of the small bowel in the protein content of the gut comes from the experiments of Nasset, who showed that the amino acid composition of the small intestine was similar in fasting and fed animals (14).

Function of Intestinal Secretions in Man

Present evidence suggests that the major function of intestinal secretions is that of a lubricant rather than a buffer or neutralizing substance (7). While the role of the succus entericus has been reduced, recent studies on the pathophysiology of cholera indicate that hypersecretion occurs in this disease and may be an important factor in the genesis of diarrheal diseases (18).

References

1. Berlin, J. D. The localization of acid mucopolysaccharides in the Golgi complex of intestinal goblet cells. *J. Cell. Biol.* **32:** 760–766, 1967.
2. Cooke, A. R., and M. I. Grossman. Studies on the secretion and motility of Brunner's gland pouches. *Gastroenterology* **51:** 506–514, 1966.
3. Cooke, A. R. The glands of Brunner. In: *Handbook of Physiology.* Section 6: Alimentary Tract. Vol. II: Secretion. Edited by C. F. Code. Washington, D.C.: American Physiological Society, 1967, pp. 1087–1095.

4. Crabbe, P. A., and J. F. Heremans. The distribution of immunoglobulin-containing cells along the human gastrointestinal tract. *Gastroenterology* **51**: 305–316, 1966.

5. Croft, D. S., C. A. Loehry, and J. F. N. Taylor. Small bowel deoxyribonucleic acid (DNA) and cell loss from human small intestinal mucosa. *Gut* **8**: 630–631, 1967.

6. Florey, H. W. Electron microscopic observations on goblet cells of the rat's colon. *Quart. J. Exp. Physiol.* **45**: 329–336, 1960.

7. Florey, H. W. The secretion and function of intestinal mucus. *Gastroenterology* **43**: 326–329, 1962.

8. Freeman, J. A. Goblet cell fine structure. *Anat. Rec.* **154**: 121–148, 1966.

9. Grossman, M. I. The glands of Brunner. *Physiol. Rev.* **38**: 675–690, 1958.

10. Jennings, M. A., and H. W. Florey. Autoradiographic observations on the mucous cells of the stomach and intestine. *Quart. J. Exp. Physiol.* **41**: 131–152, 1956.

11. Landor, J. H., P. H. Brasher, and L. R. Dragstedt. Experimental studies on the secretions of the isolated duodenum. *Arch. Surg.* **71**: 727–736, 1955.

12. Martin, B. F. The goblet cell pattern in the large intestine. *Anat. Rec.* **140**: 1–15, 1961.

13. Masson, P. L., J. F. Heremans, and C. Dive. Studies of the proteins of secretions from two villous tumors of the rectum. *Gastroenterologia* **105**: 270–282, 1966.

14. Nasset, E. S. The role of the digestive tract in protein metabolism. *Am. J. Digest. Dis.* **9**: 175–190, 1964.

15. Neutra, M., and C. P. Leblond. Synthesis of the carbohydrate of mucus in the Golgi complex as shown by electron microscope radioautography of goblet cells from rats injected with glucose-H^3. *J. Cell Biol.* **30**: 119–136, 1966.

16. Pentrila, A., and M. Lempinen. Enterochromaffin cells and 5-hydroxy-tryptamine in the human intestinal tract. *Gastroenterology* **54**: 375–381, 1968.

17. Shearman, D., and A. Muir. Observations on the secretory cycle of goblet cells. *Quart. J. Exp. Physiol.* **45**: 337–342, 1960.

18. Swallow, J. H., C. F. Code, and R. Freter. Effect of cholera toxin on water and ion fluxes in the canine bowel. *Gastroenterology* **54**: 35–40, 1968.

19. Trier, J. S. Studies of small intestinal crypt epithelium. II. Evidence for and mechanisms of secretory activity by undifferentiated crypt cells of the human small intestine. *Gastroenterology* **47**: 480–495, 1964.

20. Trier, J. S. Morphology of the epithelium of the small intestine. In: *Handbook of Physiology*. Section 6: Alimentary Tract. Vol. III: Absorption. Edited by C. F. Code. Washington, D.C.: American Physiological Society, 1967, pp. 1125–1175.

21. Trier, J. S., V. Lorenzonn, and K. Groehler. Pattern of secretion of Paneth cells of the small intestine of mice. *Gastroenterology* **53**: 240–249, 1967.

22. Wright, R. D., M. D. Jennings, H. W. Florey, and R. Lium. The influence of nerves and drugs on secretion by the small intestine and an investigation of the enzymes in intestinal juice. *Quart. J. Exp. Physiol.* **30**: 73–120, 1940.

Digestion

DURING MUCH OF THE ERA OF PHYSIOLOGIC experimentation, the term *digestion* has been used as synonymous with the total function of the gastrointestinal tract. More recently it has been restricted to the process by which the macro-molecules of the diet were broken down to small components which could enter the intestinal mucosa. The term *absorption* was used to describe pene-tration of the intestinal membrane. Digestion was considered to occur in the lumen of the gut where the dietary constituents were mixed with secretions from the digestive glands. It was realized that many of the digestive activities attributed to the succus entericus were the result of enzymes contained within epithelial cells shed into the lumen of the gut during cell renewal. Now electron microscopy and microdissection techniques are showing that the distinction among activities in the lumen, on the surface of the cell, within the cell membrane, and indeed just inside the cell membrane is becoming increasingly difficult. However, there remain advantages in considering those events which take place within the lumen of the intestinal tract in a gross sense, and digestion will be considered from that point of view.

Intraluminal digestion begins in the oral cavity. The principal reaction involves salivary amylase and dietary starch. Since the two remain in contact for such a short period in the mouth, most of the hydrolysis of starch occurs in the stomach. Although the pH of gastric content in man is usually unfavor-able to the reaction, the interior of a swallowed food bolus may retain an alkaline pH for some time and permit digestion to continue. Natural starch is a mixture of unbranched amylose and branching amylopectin. Salivary amylase acts to split both to maltose and glucose in a ratio of about 4 to

1. Dextrins are formed during the hydrolysis of amylopectin. The absence of amylase activity in the saliva of dogs or cats suggests that the enzyme is not of fundamental importance in digestion.

Digestion in the stomach continues with hydrolysis of short- and medium-chain triglycerides by gastric lipases and the splitting of peptide linkages in proteins by pepsin and gastricsin. As a result of the grinding activity of the pyloric antrum, gastric content is transformed into a semiliquid mass, the chyme. Osmolarity and temperature are usually brought into equilibrium with body fluids.

With the passage of gastric content into the duodenum, the essential features of digestion begin. Bile is released from the gallbladder and pancreatic juice from the pancreas, and absorptive processes may begin. Much of the recent studies of digestion has been based upon sampling intestinal content through fine-bore plastic tubes or perfusing segments of intestine and sampling at the distal end. The pathologist's description of the intestine at death is not helpful under these circumstances. Measurements with small tubes indicate that the distance from the nose to the pylorus is about 65 cm, nose to ligament of Treitz 90 cm, and nose to ileocecal valve 350 cm (13).

During the past several years, Crane in the United States and Ugolev in the USSR have presented evidence that digestive enzymes were localized to the surface of the membrane of intestinal epithelial cells (23,30). Crane has recently extended this concept to include the microvilli and their covering of glycocalyx or fuzzy coat as a digestive-absorption functional complex (4). The digestive enzymes entangled in the glycocalyx or attached to the surface of the microvilli act on the appropriate substrate which is then available for transport into the cell.

Smyth considers that food substances may come into contact with intracellular enzymes within epithelial cells shed into the lumen by diffusion. In other situations, the digestion products resulting from enzymes on the surface of cells may diffuse back into the lumen as well as enter the cells (28).

In man, important information came from sampling of intestinal content after meals. Using a liquid meal, Borgstrom et al. found that absorption of carbohydrate was complete in the upper small intestine, but the activity of invertase rose in the content of the distal intestine. They also noted that the amylase in 1 ml of intestinal content could digest 1 gm of starch per hour at 37°C, while the invertase activity could digest less than 0.02 gm of saccharide. They concluded that the enzymes of the succus entericus were of no importance from the absorption of disaccharides (2). Pancreatic trypsin and chymotrypsin activity gradually declined from the proximal jejunum to the ileum, presumably as a result of digestion of the enzymes. The pH rose from about 6 in the duodenum to 8 in the ileum. The meal contained 30 gm of triglyceride which combined with approximately 20 per cent its weight of bile acids and 2.5 to 5 per cent lysolecithin.

Solid meals can be used in a similar fashion. Fordtran and Locklear compared a steak meal having an osmolarity of 232 mOsm/kg with a milk and doughnuts meal with an osmolarity of 630 mOsm/kg (10). The latter meal reached isotonicity at about a depth of 200 cm. With the steak meal, the concentration of an inert marker rose to a maximum at a depth of 300 cm. Sodium and chloride concentrations reached their peaks at about 150 cm, while potassium fell to a plateau at this level.

Digestion of Carbohydrates

Disaccharidase activity is located in the intestinal brush border (23). A variety have been found in man, including a sucrase, lactase, and maltase (5). The sucrase or invertase activity of human intestinal content is low and cannot account for the digestion observed in a perfused segment of intestine (11). Hydrolysis was more rapid in the jejunum than in the ileum. Glucose and fructose appeared within the lumen, presumably as a result of the action of the disaccharidase on the brush border (24). Deren et al. found that a carbo-hydrate-rich diet fed to rats after a three-day fast led to a twofold increase in total intestinal sucrase and sucrase-specific activity (7). Most mucosal disaccharidases were present in infants under six months of age, but the diges-tion of amylopectin in this age group was decreased with a resulting accumu-lation of dextrins. The reduced hydrolysis of starch was the result of low levels of amylase activity (1).

Digestion of Proteins

The pancreas produces a bewildering array of endopeptidases and exo-peptidases (25). Using drainage from ileostomies, Goldberg et al. calculated that two thirds of the digestion of protein to acid-soluble peptides was the result of the action of trypsin and chymotrypsin (12). There was no contribu-tion by the small intestinal epithelium. Perfusion of the duodenal loop in man with a gelatin solution resulted in hydrolysis of 63 to 84 per cent of the pro-tein (3).

Smyth found that peptides disappeared into intestinal epithelium in excess of that accounted for by peptidase activity in the lumen. Some of the amino acids pass back into the lumen. The question of absorption of dipeptides remains unsolved.

As in the case of disaccharidases, a variety of peptidases have been found in the brush border (31). Lindberg reported five dipeptidases in the mucosa of adult humans. Activity was high in the jejunum and ileum but low in the stomach, colon, and proximal duodenum (20). Later he reported nine dipep-tidases in biopsies from 22 patients (21). Comparison of the properties of dipeptidases from intestinal mucosa with those of other tissues showed no essential differences (18). Human intestinal juice from the jejunum showed activity for only dipeptidase; L-analyl-L-proline peptidase. Juice from the ileum contained two others. In one instance, activity in the juice was unrelated to that in the mucosa (19).

Digestion of Fat

The normal digestion of fat involves the action of bile salts, phospholipids, and pancreatic lipase. Pancreatic lipase acts specifically on triglycerides to produce the 2-monoglyceride (20). The reaction is irreversible. Pancreatic lipase acts at the interface between oil droplet of the triglyceride emulsion and the surrounding water phase. The lipase may be attached to the glycocalyx of the microvilli. Formation of an emulsion may be considered the first phase of the digestion of fat (6). Lecithin is also attacked by pancreatic lipase with the formation of monoglyceride (14).

Sampling of intestinal content after a fatty meal showed four phases—an aqueous phase, a clear phase, containing lipid, an oily phase, and sediment. Dowse and colleagues sampled a jejunal fistula in two dogs and found that the clear phase contained 42 to 59 per cent fatty acid and 5 to 16 per cent monoglyceride. Hofmann and Borgstrom compared the clear and oily phases of intestinal content in man after a fatty meal (15). They found that the heavier clear phase contained fatty acid and monoglyceride, while the oily layer on the surface contained more diglyceride and triglyceride. Ordinarily the sediment contains little lipid (26). These experiments led to the suggestion that the lipid in the clear phase might be in the form of micelles (16). Since then, much effort has been expended on the study of micelles and their role in the digestion of fat. Essentially micelles are molecular aggregates involving, in this case, monoglycerides, bile salts, cholesterol, and phospholipids. Figure 8–1 (A) shows a diagrammatic representation of micelles (27). The water-soluble portions of the bile salt and lecithin molecules protrude into the aqueous phase, while the cholesterol and lipid soluble portions of the other molecules are contained in the interior. Only the bile salts are in equilibrium with molecules in the aqueous phase surrounding the micelle. A similar model could be constructed with monoglyceride rather than cholesterol. (Fig. 8-1B) Among the important characteristics of micelles is their dependence upon temperature and concentration of the constituents (17). Tamesue and Juniper found that the critical micellar concentrations for human gallbladder bile was 1.3 to 1.6 mM/L for total bile acids and 0.5 mM for phospholipids (29). The result of the formation of monoglyceride micelles is a water-soluble aggregate on the surface which can then attach to the absorptive cell surface.

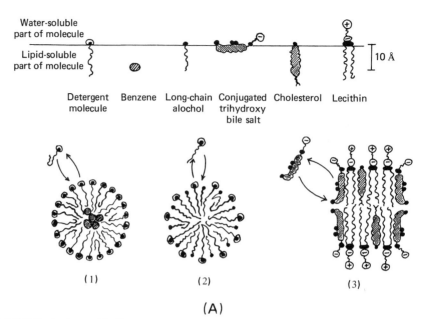

FIGURE 8-1.   (A) The several types of lipid molecules and the cross-sectional arrangement of these molecules in three types of mixed micelles are represented diagrammatically. *Wavy lines:* the lipid-soluble hydrocarbon chain part of the molecule; *Shaded area:* the lipid-soluble cyclic hydrocarbon part of the molecule; ⊙ the polar head of the detergent molecule; • OH groups or ester groups, as the case may be; ⊕ and ⊖ the positively and negatively charged ionic polar groups. The molecules have been depicted so that their water-soluble parts lie above the line and their fat-soluble parts below the line. Although the polar and nonpolar regions of most amphipathic substances are at opposite ends of the long axis of the molecule, it can be seen that bile salt is peculiar in that the lipophilic part of the ring is confined to one side, the other side being hydrophilic and spiked with several OH groups. This peculiar structure accounts for many of the properties of bile salts divergent from ordinary detergents. The lower part of (A) represents the cross section of three mixed micelles. (1) A mixed micelle of nonpolar benzene held in solution by detergent. The benzene molecules lie in the lipid center of the micelle. Only the detergent molecules are in equilibrium with the molecules in the surrounding aqueous medium. (2) A mixed micelle of insoluble amphipath (long chain alcohol) and detergent. The alcohol with its OH group in the aqueous medium interdigitates with the detergent. Again, only the detergent molecules are in equilibrium with the molecules in the surrounding aqueous medium. (3) A mixed micelle of bile salt, lecithin, and cholesterol. The proposed structure of this mixed micelle is a cylinder-shaped bimolecular disk of lecithin and cholesterol stabilized on its hydrophobic surface by the bile salts. Note that the entire surface of this micelle, like other micelles, is hydrophilic, and that the lipophilic parts of the molecules are in the interior of the micelle. Only the bile salts are in equilibrium with molecules in the aqueous medium surrounding the micelle. Since the height of the micelle is very close to its diameter, this micelle would appear spherical by most physiochemical methods. (From D. M. Small: *Gastroenterology* **52:** 609, ©️ 1967, The Williams & Wilkins Co., Baltimore, Md. 21202, U.S.A.)

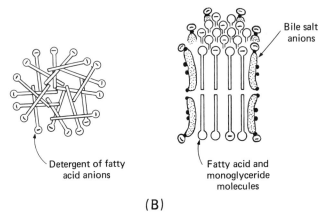

Bile salt
anions

Detergent of fatty
acid anions

Fatty acid and
monoglyceride
molecules

(B)

FIGURE 8-1.   (B) The probable molecular arrangement of a typical soap or anionic detergent (*left*) is contrasted to a proposed model for the bile salt-polar lipid micelle (*right*). A cross section of micelle is shown: the aggregate on the left is spherical; that on the right, disk shaped. Bound counter-ions, although present, are not shown, nor is the rapid exchange of molecules presumed to occur between those of the micelle and the much smaller fraction in true solution. The center of the micelle is composed of liquid paraffin chains of the polar lipid, and these hydrocarbon chains are chiefly responsible for the solvent capacity of the bile salt-polar lipid micelle. The model on the right was proposed by Small for the bile salt-polar lecithin systems. The bile salts serve as adsorbed, dispersing agents for lipids capable of spontaneously forming large hydrated bimolecular leaflets in water. Bile salts transform these large, lamellar, weakly charged aggregates into small, charged disks or spheres. With higher ratios of polar lipid to bile salt, the aggregate will elongate to a larger disk of bimolecular thickness (*right*). (From A. F. Hofmann, *Medium Chain Triglycerides,* edited by J. R. Senior, Philadelphia: University of Pennsylvania Press, 1968, pp. 9–19.)

Digestion in Man

Digestion begins through the action of hydrolytic enzymes in the digestive secretions but is completed by enzymes resting in the brush border of the small intestinal surface epithelial cells. The digestion of starch is carried to the level of glucose, and sucrose is hydrolyzed to glucose and fructose. Proteins are broken down to amino acids. Dietary triglycerides form emulsions where they are hydrolyzed to monoglycerides by pancreatic lipase. The monoglycerides enter into micelles together with bile salts and phospholipids. In this form they attach to intestinal epithelial cells.

Pathophysiology

Incomplete digestion can be expected to occur in the absence of pancreatic juice or bile. Intestinal content can be assayed for lipolytic activity, bile salt concentration, and micelle formation. Diffuse pancreatic disease, interruption of the enterohepatic circulation (32), or qualitative changes in bile salts due to bacterial action in blind intestinal loops may lead to maldigestion of fat. Vagotomy also produces abnormal fat digestion, but the mechanism is not clear (9).

References

1. Aurrichio, S., D. Della Pietra, and A. Vegnente. Studies on intestinal digestion of starch in man. II. Intestinal hydrolysis of amylopectin in infants and children. *Pediatrics* **39**: 853–862, 1967.

2. Borgstrom, B., A. Dahlquist, G. Lundh, and J. Sjovall. Studies of intestinal digestion and absorption in the human. *J. Clin. Invest.* **36**: 1521–1536, 1957.

3. Cerda, J. J., F. P. Brooks, and D. J. Prockop. Intraduodenal hydrolysis of gelatin as a measure of protein digestion in normal subjects and in patients with malabsorption syndrome. *Gastroenterology* **54**: 358–365, 1968.

4. Crane, R. K. A perspective of digestion-absorption function—1968. Proc. Intern. Union Physiol Sci. Vol. VI. XXIV Intern. Congress. Washington, D.C., 1968, pp. 103–104.

5. Dahlquist, A., S. Aurrichio, G. Semenza, and A. Prader. Human intestinal disaccharidases and hereditary disaccharide intolerance. The hydrolysis of sucrose, isomaltose, palatinose (isomaltulose) and a 1,6-α-oligosaccharide (isomalto-oligosaccharide) preparation. *J. Clin. Invest.* **42**: 556–562, 1963.

6. Dawson, A. M. Bile salts and fat absorption. *Gut* **8**: 1–3, 1967.

7. Deren, J. J., S. A. Broitman, and N. Zamcheck. Effect of diet upon intestinal disaccharidases and disaccharide absorption. *J. Clin. Invest.* **46**: 186–195, 1967.

8. Dowse, C. M., J. A. Saunders, and B. Schofield. The composition of lipid from jejunal contents of the dog after a fatty meal. *J. Physiol.* **134**: 515–526, 1956.

9. Fields, M., and H. L. Duthie. Effect of vagotomy on intraluminal digestion of fat in man. *Gut* **6**: 301–310, 1965.

10. Fordtran, J. S., and T. W. Locklear. Ionic constituents and osmolarities of gastric and small intestinal fluids after eating. *Am. J. Dig. Dis.* **11**: 503–521, 1966.

11. Gray, G. M., and F. J. Inglefinger. Intestinal absorption of sucrose in man: The site of hydrolysis and absorption. *J. Clin. Invest.* **44**: 390–398, 1965.

12. Goldberg, D. M., R. R. McAllister, and A. D. Roy. Studies on human intestinal proteolysis. *Scand. J. Gastroenterol.* **3**: 193–201, 1968.

13. Hirsch, J., E. H. Ahrens, Jr., and D. H. Blankenhorn. Measurement of human intestinal length in vivo and some causes of variation. *Gastroenterology* **31**: 274–284, 1956.

14. Hofmann, A. F., and B. Borgstrom. Hydrolysis of long-chain monoglycerides in micellar solution by pancreatic lipase. *Biochim. Biophys. Acta* **70**: 317–331, 1963.

15. Hofmann, A. F., and B. Borgstrom. The intraluminal phase of fat digestion in man: The lipid content of the micellar and oil phases of intestinal content obtained during fat digestion and absorption. *J. Clin. Invest.* **43**: 247–257, 1964.

16. Hofmann, A. F. A physicochemical approach to the intraluminal phase of fat absorption. *Gastroenterology* **50**: 56–64, 1966.

17. Hofmann, A. F. Intraluminal factors in the absorption of glycerides. In: *Medium Chain Triglycerides*, edited by J. R. Senior. Philadelphia: University of Pennsylvania Press. 1968, pp. 9–19.
18. Josefsson, L., O. Noren, and H. Sjostrom. Comparison of dipeptidase activity in different tissues of the pig. *Acta Physiol. Scand.* **72:** 108–114, 1968.
19. Josefsson, L., T. Lindberg, and L. Ojesjo. Intestinal dipeptidases. Dipeptidase activities in human intestinal juice. *Scand. J. Gastroent.* **3:** 207–210, 1968.
20. Lindberg, T. Intestinal dipeptidases. Dipeptidase activity in the mucosa of the gastrointestinal tract of the adult human. *Acta Physiol. Scand.* **66:** 437–443, 1966.
21. Lindberg, T., A. Norden, and L. Josefsson. Intestinal dipeptidases. Dipeptidase activities in small intestinal biopsy specimens from a clinical material. *Scand. J. Gastroent.* **3:** 177–182, 1968.
22. Mattson, F. H., and L. W. Beck. The specificity of pancreatic lipase for the primary hydroxyl groups of glycerides. *J. Biol. Chem.* **219:** 735–740, 1956.
23. Miller, D., and R. K. Crane. The digestive function of the epithelium of the small intestine. I. An intracellular locus of disaccharide and sugar phosphate ester hydrolysis. *Biochim. Biophys. Acta* **52:** 281–293, 1961.
24. Nadirova, T. Ya, V. A. Timofeev, and A. M. Ugolev. Localization of the invertase activity in the cells of the small intestines of albino rats. *Bull. Exp. Biol. Med.* **59:** 250–253, 1965 (English transl.).
25. Neurath, H. Protein-digesting enzymes. *Sci. Amer.* **211:** 68–79, 1964.
26. Simmonds, W. J., A. F. Hofmann, and E. Theodore. Absorption of cholesterol from a micellar solution: Intestinal perfusion studies in man. *J. Clin. Invest.* **46:** 874–890, 1967.
27. Small, D. M. Physicochemical studies of cholesterol gallstone formation. *Gastroenterology* **52:** 607–610, 1967.
28. Smyth, D. H. Intestinal absorption. In: *Recent Advances in Physiology.* Edited by R. Creese (8th ed.). Boston: Little, Brown & Co., 1963, pp. 36–68.
29. Tamesue, N., and K. Juniper. Concentrations of bile salts at the critical micellar concentration of human gall bladder bile. *Gastroenterology* **52:** 473–479, 1967.
30. Ugolev, A. M. Membrane (contact) digestion. *Physiol. Rev.* **45:** 555–595, 1965.
31. Ugolev, A. M. Hydrolysis of dipeptides in cells of the small intestine. *Nature* **212:** 859–860, 1966.
32. Van Deest, B. W., J. S. Fordtran, S. G. Morawski, and J. D. Wilson. Bile salt and micellar fat concentration in proximal small bowel contents of iliectomy patients. *J. Clin. Invest.* **47:** 1314–1324, 1968.

Absorption

ABSORPTION IS THE MAJOR FUNCTION of the gastrointestinal tract. To the casual observer, it might appear that the small intestine exerts little control over absorption. Carbohydrate, protein, and fat are absorbed in sufficient quantities even after extensive resections, and significant degrees of malabsorption are uncommon in general medical practice. However, recent investigations indicate that this may not be the case. The intestine plays a central role in the control of absorption and metabolism of iron and cholesterol. There is evidence that the absorption of carbohydrate may be subject to controlling influences originating in part outside the intestine.

A brief survey of the literature shows that this area of gastrointestinal physiology has become the most active research interest in the field. In 1921, Samuel Goldschmidt, writing in the first volume of *Physiological Reviews*, stated that the absorption of substances from the intestine was the result of physicochemical laws, particularly osmotic gradients (*61*). Since then, the phenomenon of active transport, possibly mediated by carriers in the cell membrane, has become a major concept in the mechanism of absorption. There have been many reviews of the subject, including the following: references *11, 140, 155, 157, 159.*

The Structural Basis of Absorption

The wall of the intestinal tube can be divided into the mucosa and serosa, separated by a submucosa, muscularis mucosae, and muscularis propria. In the small intestine, the muscularis propria is divided into an inner circular and outer longitudinal layer. This is shown diagrammatically in Figure 9-1. For autonomic control, it is important to note the two nervous plexuses—the myenteric (Auerbach), lying between the two layers of the muscularis propria, and the submucosal (Meissner), lying in the submucosa. Despite years of study, the anatomic relationship of these ganglion cells to the extrinsic nerves and to smooth muscle remain uncertain.

The mucosa itself is an extremely interesting tissue. It has one of the more

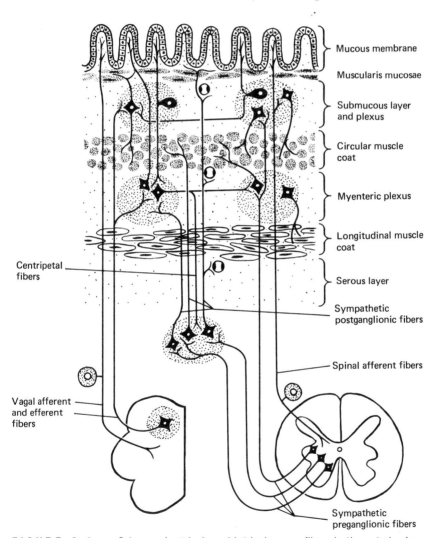

FIGURE 9-1. Schema of extrinsic and intrinsic nerve fibers in the enteric plexus. (From Schofield. *International Review of General and Experimental Zoology.* Edited by W. J. L. Felts and R. J. Harrison, New York: Academic Press, 1968.)

rapid turnover rates of cells in the body, and its capacity for protein synthesis is also very high. The surface is thrown into many fingerlike projections or villi which greatly increase the surface area for absorption. Hendrix and his associates made reconstructions of the mucosa which show the villi arising like the cone of a South Pacific atoll from the surrounding crypts. Figure 9-2 is taken from their paper (22).

The villi decrease in number from jejunum to ileum with a corresponding

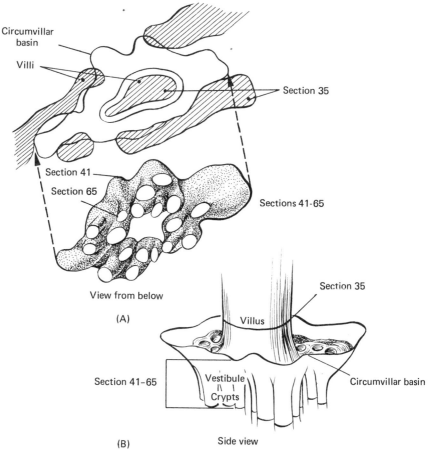

FIGURE 9-2. This diagram represents the basement membrane rather than the luminal surface of the epithelium. (A) shows the reconstruction as viewed from below; (B) shows the same reconstruction as viewed from the side. At the level of section 65, 10 crypts of Lieberkuhn surround a villus core. At the level of section 41, the crypts have coalesced to form the "circumvillar basin" [represented by solid line in upper half of (A)]. At the level of section 35 the "circumvillar basins" have intercommunicated to form the intervillous space. The cross-hatched areas show the cross section of the villi at this level. (From A. E. Cocco, M. J. Dohrmann, and T. R. Hendrix: *Gastroenterology* **51**: 24–31, ⓒ 1966, The Williams & Wilkins Co., Baltimore, Md. 21202, U.S.A.)

decrease in surface area. On the other hand, collections of lymphocytes in follicles grow more prominent, forming the Peyer's patches of the ileum.

The light microscopic view of the small intestine is dominated by the presence of villi. It is of critical importance that the sections be cut perpendicular to the surface in order to show their fingerlike projections; otherwise the surface may appear flattened. The surface of the villi is covered primarily by tall columnar cells with occasional goblet cells, Paneth cells, and argentaffin cells (146). The submucosa contains connective tissue cells, macrophages, lymphocytes, and plasma cells (116).

The ultrastructure of the intestinal epithelium, as seen with the electron microscope, shows cells with the characteristics of great metabolic activity. Probably the most striking feature is the microvilli. These fingerlike projections extend from the luminal surface, as seen in Figure 9-3. Trier stated that they increase the surface area by a factor of 14- to 39-fold over a flat surface (146). Figure 9-4 shows a diagram of the microvillous area in more detail. The "fuzz" or glycocalyx is a mucoproteinaceous coat closely attached to the surface of the microvilli.

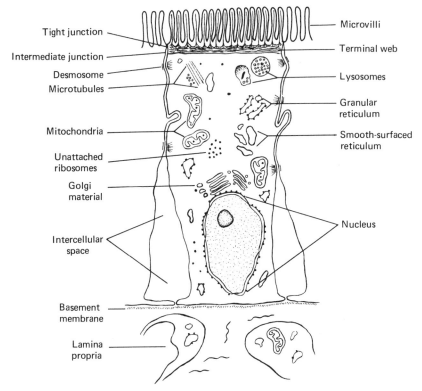

Tight junction
Microvilli
Intermediate junction
Terminal web
Desmosome
Microtubules
Lysosomes
Granular reticulum
Mitochondria
Smooth-surfaced reticulum
Unattached ribosomes
Golgi material
Intercellular space
Nucleus
Basement membrane
Lamina propria

FIGURE 9-3.   Schematic diagram of the interstinal absorptive cell. (From J. S. Trier and C. E. Rubin. *Gastroenterology* **49**: 574–603, © 1965. The Williams & Wilkins Co., Baltimore, Md. 21202, U.S.A.)

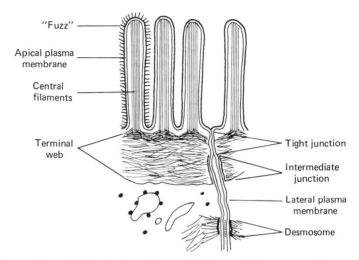

"Fuzz"

Apical plasma membrane

Central filaments

Terminal web

Tight junction

Intermediate junction

Lateral plasma membrane

Desmosome

FIGURE 9-4.   Schematic illustration of the specializations of the apical cytoplasm of the plasma membrane of intestinal absorptive cells. (From J. S. Trier and C. E. Rubin. *Gastroenterology* **49:** 574–603, © 1965, The Williams & Wilkins Co., Baltimore, Md. 21202, U.S.A.)

Other important features of the ultrastructure are the tight junctions binding the adjacent cells together in their apical portions and the intercellular spaces along the lateral borders of the cells. The terminal web below the microvilli consists of rather dense tissue and may act as a barrier. The prominent rough endoplasmic reticulum suggests abundant protein synthesis.

The flattening of the villi, which occurs with increasing distance from the pylorus, suggests that functional differences may also occur. In general, the proximal small intestine appears to be the more active site of absorption for many nutrients. Some such as calcium, magnesium, and iron are absorbed from the duodenum, possibly because this is the first area exposed. The proximal jejunum is the major absorptive site for glucose, thiamine, riboflavin, pyridoxine, folic acid, and vitamin C. Fat and protein are also absorbed from the jejunum but at sites somewhat more distal than glucose. The ileum seems to possess unique absorptive mechanisms for the transport of vitamin B_{12} and bile salts (*12,46*). It is important to distinguish between sites of greatest absorption as determined with in vitro segments and under in vivo conditions.

Cell Renewal in the Intestinal Mucosa

The rate of cell renewal in the mucosa is a matter of great functional significance. The presence of occasional mitotic figures in cells lining the intestinal crypts had been known for many years, but it was the use of tritiated thymidine as an isotopic tracer of DNA synthesis that made it possible to study this problem quantitatively. By means of autoradiographs, it is possible to construct the following cycle. Cells that are synthesizing DNA incorporate the label into the molecule which then appears as a grain on the autoradiograph. This is the S phase of synthesis. It is followed by a period of preparation, the G_2 phase of postsynthesis or premitosis. In man, the generation time for the proliferating cells of the intestinal crypts is about 24 hours. Figure 9-5 illustrates the cycle.

Using such techniques, surface epithelial cells have been traced from the depths of the crypts to the tips of the villi where they are shed into the lumen (97). In man, it takes about five to seven days for cells of the duodenal or jejunal crypts to complete this journey. Paneth cells and enterochromaffin cells apparently turn over much more slowly.

Since the intestinal mucosa of the adult retains a rather uniform cell population, the system should be regulated. According to Munro, mucosal shedding from the intestine releases 250 gm/day, of which 50 gm is protein (107). Protein-deficient diets and x-radiation reduce the rate of intestinal DNA synthesis. The factors determining whether a given cell continues to pass through the synthetic cycle or enters a prolonged inactive phase are unknown. Cairnie et al. suggest that cells in the crypts can be divided into two types—a proliferative cell, which gives rise to two daughter cells; and another cell whose daughter cells differentiate. Under circumstances leading to increased cell production, fewer cells differentiate (16). Using cell mitosis as an index, Bejar et al. found no evidence that vagotomy influenced cell turnover in man (10).

The behavior of the intestinal mucosa has great significance in disease. Atrophic lesions of the mucosa may result either from arrested development and prolonged generation times or from excessive shedding of cells in the

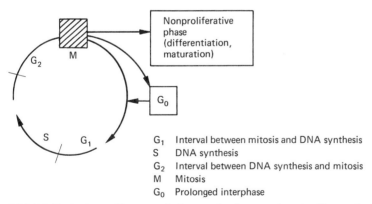

G_1 Interval between mitosis and DNA synthesis
S   DNA synthesis
G_2 Interval between DNA synthesis and mitosis
M   Mitosis
G_0 Prolonged interphase

FIGURE 9-5. Diagram of phases of cell renewal cycle. Phases G_1 (postmitotic, presynthetic), S (DNA synthesis), G_2 (postsynthetic, premitotic), and M (mitosis) constiute the cycle. Phase G_0 indicates prolonged interphase, containing fertile cells, not proliferating. Cells enter a nonproliferative phase during differentiation and maturations. (From M. Lipkin, *Fed. Proc.* **24:** 11, 1965.)

presence of a normal generation time. Autoimmune reactions or enzymatic defects might be expected to interfere with synthesis (29).

Growth and Adaptation

The human small intestine in the early stages of development is lined by a stratified epithelium of two to four layers. The duodenal lumen is occluded at the 16-mm stage and complete patency is not reestablished until the 24-mm length is reached (35). The muscularis mucosae does not appear in the rat until the eighth day postpartum, and the microvilli of the duodenum and jejunum do not reach the adult appearance until just before weaning. The 30-day embryo in the rabbit showed filling of the apical cytoplasm of the surface epithelial cells of the ileum with thick-walled membraneous vesicles. This may be related to the absorption of immunoglobulins at this stage. Adrenocortical hormones induce more rapid differentiation of the epithelial cells, and hypophysectomy retards maturation.

During the last three months of fetal life there is a rapid increase in the development of villi and microvilli. In general the morphologic changes are accompanied by increased absorption of sugar and amino acids. However, some transport systems show an asynchronous development, suggesting qualitative changes in the brush border. The human jejunum and ileum by the twelfth to fifteenth week of gestation showed electrogenic hexose and amino acid transfer mechanisms (90).

The adaptive changes in brush border enzymes have been noted in the chapter on digestion. The response of the remaining intestine to resection of large portions of small intestine is also of interest. Increases in absorption of glucose by intestinal loops occurred in humans after intestinal resection (47). Feeding an inert substance such as kaolin increased the absorptive capacity for glucose and water in rats. There was no significant change in surface area, but the activity of leucine aminopeptidase and several dehydrogenases increased. Hyperphagia, lactation, and pregnancy produced dilatation and hypertrophy of the small intestine. Semistarvation in rats was followed in a few days by a striking increase in the absorption of l-histidine and of glucose. Return to a normal diet resulted in normal absorption within a few days (83).

Properties of the Small Intestine

The permeability of the small intestinal mucosa can be determined by application of the same principles used in the circulation. Pore size in the human jejunum has been estimated at 7 to 9 Å, compared to 3 to 4 in the ileum (51). In order to account for experimental results, it was necessary to assume that jejunal cell pores were either fewer in number or longer in length, or both, than in the ileum.

Electrical potential differences can be recorded across the intestinal wall and the cell membranes of the epithelial cells. In the rat, the potential across isolated segments of small intestine fell from 8 mv in the jejunum to 4 in the ileum (21). The mucosa was negative with respect to the serosa. Stripping off the muscularis made little difference, so that the potential seemed to arise within the mucosa (9). The transmural potential was increased in the presence of glucose and other hexoses which are actively transported. Amino acids also increase the transmural potential.

The transmembrane potential of epithelial cells of the intestine range from 7 to 25 mv, with the inside negative to the outside. The potential difference with respect to the luminal surface is greater across the serosal membrane and opposite in polarity to that across the apical membrane. The addition of glucose or alanine led to a rise in the PD across the serosal cell membrane rather than the luminal membrane of the epithelial cell (9). Using an elegant intracellular technique, Lowenstein et al. showed that ions passed quite freely between epithelial cells of the salivary glands, but not across the surface facing the lumen (99). The precise relationship between the PD across the mucosa and absorption is unknown (89).

Techniques for the Study of Absorption

Absorption has been studied by both in vitro and in vivo techniques. Fisher and Parsons devised an in vitro technique in which a segment of rat intestine was mounted in such a fashion that the lumen was perfused with one solution, while another solution circulated around the outside of the segment (Figure 9-6). With this preparation they were able to show transport of glucose against a concentration gradient. Wilson and Wiseman later reported that the hamster intestine could be everted and cut into segments that would transport material from a solution bathing the mucosa into the serosal cavity, as shown in Figure 9-7. The small volume of the serosal compartment made it easier to detect transfer of small amounts of substance (115).

FIGURE 9-6.   Circulation unit for investigating absorption by intestine in vitro. ▶ R and B: water-jacketed reservoir. G_1 and G_2: gas lifts. The intestinal segment is suspended on the cannulas C_1 and C_2 and immersed in the serosal fluid I contained in reservoir B. The mucosal fluid circuit flows from R through the segment and is returned to R via J. Note that the serosal fluid, I, is also recirculated through a system including the gas lift G. A: air condenser; $h_0 = 40$ cm, $h_1 = 35$ cm, d is variable and usually between 10 and 35cm distention pressure. Pressure differential in system which determines flow rate in lumen circuit is $(h_1 - \Phi h_0)$ cm of saline, where Φ is fraction of length of liquid column in J which is occupied by liquid. (From R. B. Fisher and D. S. Parsons. J. Physiol. London 110: 37, 1949.)

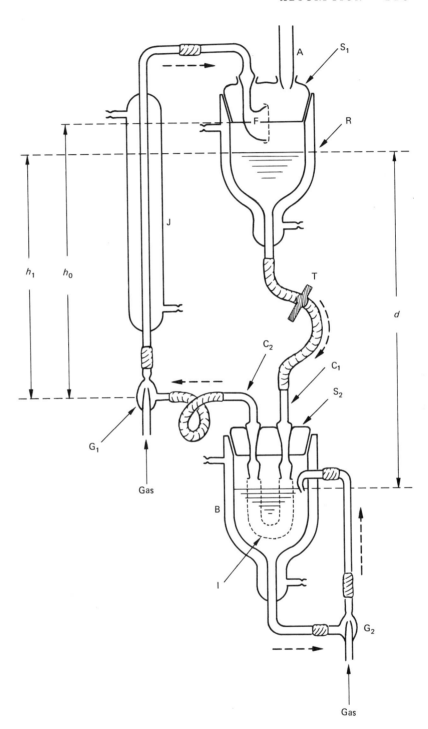

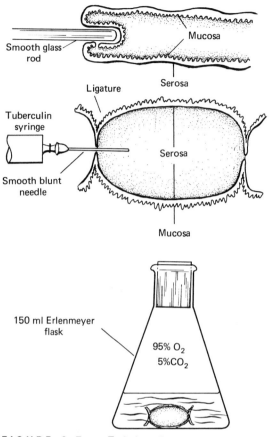

FIGURE 9-7. Technique for preparation of everted sacs. *Top:* one end of an intestinal segment is invaginated over a glass rod; the segment is then rolled over the invaginated end. When the invaginated end appears at the lumen of the distal end of the intestine, eversion is completed by gently rolling the intestinal wall over on itself while on the glass rod. *Middle:* everted segment, tied off at right-hand end, is filled from a tuberculin syringe at left-hand end. A blunt needle attached to the syringe is passed through the loose ligature which is then pulled tightly over the needle, the appropriate volume of fluid is injected and the needle then withdrawn. *Bottom:* sac is incubated in a flask containing a suitable volume of incubation medium in equilibrium with an appropriate gas mixture, in this case, O_2 and CO_2. (From G. Wiseman. In: *Methods in Medical Research,* Vol. 9. Edited by J. H. Quastel. Copyright © 1961. Chicago: Year Book Medical Publisher, Inc. Used by permission of the Year Book Medical Publishers.)

Crane has developed microdissection techniques that permit the isolation of microvilli and brush borders. This has permitted the study of absorption as an intracellular process. Slices of intestine can be used to study uptake of material from solutions.

While in vitro techniques permit the study of transport in the absence of confusing variables, mucosal to serosal transport may differ significantly from the usual mucosal to blood or lymph movement. Oxygenation preserves histologic normality but only for limited periods, and more subtle changes may affect the results.

For the study of absorption in vivo, the most popular technique has been the perfusion of intestinal loops either in the open abdomen in acute experiments or by means of fistulas in chronic animals. A further refinement of technique has been to cannulate the vascular and lymphatic supply to the loop.

In man, passage of a double-lumen tube into a segment of intestine permitted perfusion of a fluid into the proximal end of the loop and aspiration at the distal end. In order to determine net movement of water and solutes from the perfusate, it is necessary to include a marker that is neither digested nor absorbed during the perfusion. The most popular marker is polyethyleneglycol (PEG), but other agents that can be measured more easily have been used (54,121). Fordtran and Inglefinger refer to this technique as "perfusion-marker" technique. A similar approach can be used with a meal (53). A basic assumption of the perfusion-marker technique is that the marker and test substances are uniformly distributed in the same phase. Aspiration of the perfusate occurs at an uneven rate, so that the method is not suitable for short-term changes. Figure 9-8 shows a diagram of such a method with an added feature of a third lumen, permitting aspiration at two levels of the intestine (25).

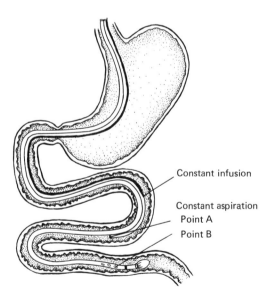

Constant infusion

Constant aspiration
Point A
Point B

FIGURE 9-8. Diagram of triple-lumen tube positioned in the intestine. (From H. Cooper, R. Levitan, F. S. Fordtran, and F. J. Inglefinger. *Gastroenterology* **50:** 1–7, © 1966, The Williams & Wilkins Co., Baltimore, Md. 21202, U.S.A.)

Borgstrom et al. used a single aspiration tip after a liquid meal including isotopically labeled substances to determine the site of absorption of food substances as they passed through the intestine. Similar studies have been made with solid meals, determining net movement of electrolytes.

Terminology of Intestinal Absorption

Students of absorption in vitro become concerned with the structure of membranes and the physicochemical principles governing membrane transport. Levin wrote that their eventual goal was to determine the amount transferred per cell and the associated changes in cellular concentration (91). Since the net flux across a membrane is the resultant of unidirectional fluxes in both directions, the latter have been referred to as mucosal-to-serosal or serosal-to-mucosal fluxes. During the process of transfer there is also uptake of the substance within the tissue itself. If the potential difference across the mucosa is reduced by an electrical current passed so as to oppose the PD, ion movement in the absence of a concentration gradient reflects an active process. The magnitude of the "short-circuit current" necessary may be an indication of the equivalents of ion transferred.

The central term in transport across membranes is *active transport*, defined most simply as movement against an electrochemical gradient. In vitro this required measurement of both concentrations across the membrane and the potential difference for electrically charged particles. It is supported further by the evidence of metabolic inhibitors or cell poisons in halting the process. The most popular hypothesis to account for the phenomenon of active transport is the presence of a carrier, usually a protein, which by binding to the substance to be transported may then move to the opposite side of the membrane and release the substance. The mobile carrier concept may require energy on the part of the cell. This would account for the requirement of energy expenditure for active transport. In some circumstances the evidence seems clear, but Curran has pointed out that what appears to be an energy-dependent process may be coupled to a general cellular metabolic process such as the extrusion of sodium rather than a unique process required for transport (32).

In vivo absorption also involves bidirectional fluxes with the additional feature of movement into blood. Code has suggested the terms *sorption* for net transport, *insorption* for lumen-to-blood movement, and *exsorption* for blood-to-lumen movement. None of these terms has been generally accepted. In order to demonstrate active transport in man, enzyme kinetics have been used to show saturation of the carrier mechanism and to determine the quantitative characteristics of the reaction. For this purpose, the reciprocal of the amount of substance perfused may be plotted against the reciprocal of the amount absorbed, the Lineweaver-Burk plot. From this the V_{max} and velocity constant, k, can be determined. While such data are suggestive, they have rarely established the presence of active transport to the satisfaction of most investigators.

The Absorption of Water and Electrolyte

The principal site of water absorption is in the small intestine. In the stomach water leaves the lumen at one tenth the rate of that in the small bowel, according to studies with heavy water in man (131). Perfusions of the human colon showed that sodium, chloride, and water were absorbed, and potassium and bicarbonate were added to the luminal content (92). The central problems in water absorption are the route of absorption and the mechanism by which it crosses the mucosa. The anatomic features of tight junctions between cells seem to make the entrance of water between cells unlikely. However, Williams found dilated intercellular spaces below the tight junctions during water absorption, suggesting that water may leave the cells by this route (153). The excessive thermodynamic demands for active transport of water and the in vitro evidence that water transport followed solute movement have made active transport of water an unpopular concept. Grim still considered pinocytosis a possible mechanism of water transport in the gallbladder, however (65). Lee and Duncan found that in rat jejunum without vascular perfusion, 85 per cent of the water absorbed was transported via the lymphatics. When the system was perfused from artery to vein, 10 to 25 per cent appeared in the lymphatics (86). Osmotic forces influence water absorption, but over a range, serosal fluid was isosmotic with fluid in the lumen whether the latter was hypertonic, isotonic, or hypotonic (87).

In vitro absorption of sodium chloride appears to be the result of active transport of sodium, with chloride following passively (135). However, a number of experiments in vivo suggest that chloride does not follow sodium in a simple fashion.

In the rat jejunum, chloride was absorbed more slowly than sodium, but in the ileum, chloride was absorbed at least as fast (114). Visscher et al. also noted "chloride impoverishment" of ileal content in dogs (148). Isolated colonic loops in dogs were filled with isotonic saline and later showed a fall in chloride concentration and a rise in bicarbonate, with the sum remaining constant (33). In man, using perfusion studies, Fordtran et al. found that in the jejunum, sodium was absorbed against a modest concentration gradient and was influenced by the presence of sugar. In the ileum, sodium was absorbed against a very steep electrochemical gradient, and absorption was not influenced by sugars or bicarbonate. They concluded that the major absorption of sodium in man was by the process of bulk flow (52).

Bicarbonate represents the other major anion in intestinal content. Hubel found evidence for a relationship between chloride absorption and the secretion of bicarbonate in loops of ileum of rats (74,75). In dogs and man, the equilibrium values for bicarbonate concentrations in intestinal content were 5 mM/L in the jejunum but 40 to 75 in the ileum (119,142). In dogs, there was a bidirectional flux in all segments, but insorption varied with the luminal concentration. Exsorption was independent of luminal concentration in the distal ileum and colon (142).

Potassium absorption appeared to occur passively in response to a concentration gradient in the Thiry-Vella loops in dogs but was actively transported into the lumen from the blood in the ileum and colon (118).

Calcium absorption involves an active transport mechanism in the proximal small intestine (129). Uphill transport occurred both at the medium-to-mucosal junction and from the mucosa to the underlying coats. The latter process was dependent upon oxidative phosphorylation and both steps require vitamin D (130). Vitamin D did not act in vitro. Parathyroidectomy reduced calcium absorption in rats in vivo (139). Schedl found that calcium was absorbed against a concentration gradient throughout the small intestine in rats. Net transport was highest in the duodenum. The gradient between lumen and tissue was uphill, but that between tissue and blood was downhill (84). In the dog, calcium was secreted in the jejunum but absorbed in the terminal ileum from luminal contents. In Thiry-Vella loops calcium was absorbed from the jejunum (134). Nordin summarized evidence that absorption of calcium involved an unknown carrier protein which was synthesized by a process requiring vitamin D (109). Supplemental magnesium fed to rats receiving at least 0.4 per cent calcium increased the absorption of calcium (20).

Iron absorption bears a number of similarities to calcium absorption. It is absorbed primarily from the proximal small intestine, and the mechanism probably involves a carrier protein (64). Under ordinary circumstances much of the dietary iron is in the form of hemoglobin. Conrad et al. found that, in man, heme was split off from globin in the lumen of the gut and absorbed as a metalloporphyrin. Substances that decreased the polymerization of heme increased the absorption of heme iron. Absorption may be controlled by the release of iron from heme within the cells or by the quantity of iron transferred to the plasma (23).

One of the main interests in iron absorption is the nature of the control mechanism which maintains the total body iron within limits, permitting the absorption of about 10 mg of iron per day. In some fashion the epithelial cells of the gut are able to accumulate iron in relation to the total body iron stores. This, in turn, limits the amount of iron that enters the cell from the lumen. Figure 9-9 shows a scheme of the control of iron absorption to account for the increase of iron absorption when the body iron stores are depleted and the reduction in absorption when the body is iron-loaded (30). It shows that mucosal iron is in equilibrium with plasma iron bound to transferrin. The amount of iron bound to transferrin depends upon the amount of iron stored as ferritin, hemoglobin iron, and iron in cellular pigments and enzymes. The

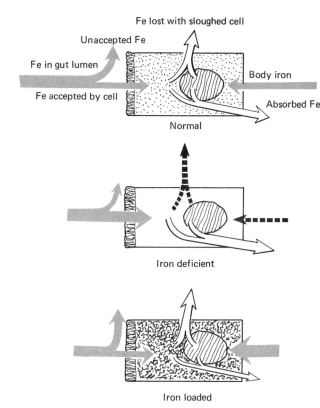

FIGURE 9-9.   A concept of control of iron absorption by the intestinal mucosa. It is predicated that iron absorption is regulated primarily through the columnar epithelium of the small intestine. In normal, iron-replete subjects the mucosal cells may contain a variable amount of iron supplied from the body store. This deposit regulates, within limits, the quantity of iron that can enter the cell from the gut lumen. After the dietary iron has entered the cell, it may proceed into the body to fulfill a requirement. Alternatively, a portion of the iron may become fixed in the epithelial cytoplasm to be lost when the cell is sloughed at the end of its lifespan. In iron-deficient subjects there appears to be little inhibition to the entrance of iron into the villous epithelial cells and no capacity to retain it. Thus dietary iron readily proceeds into the body. In ironloaded subjects the body iron incorporated in the epithelial cells is eventually lost, but during the lifespan of the cells its presence inhibits the entrance of dietary iron into the cells. (From M. E. Conrad and W. H. Crosby. *Blood* **22:** 429–440, 1963.)

iron of hemoglobin may be picked up by phagocytes that leave the circulation in the intestinal mucosa. The amount of iron in intestinal epithelial cells appears to be determined by the equilibrium state at the time the cell begins to move from the intestinal crypt to the villous tip. Electron microscopy has identified tetrahedrons of ferritin in intestinal epithelial cells. Both epithelial cells and phagocytes may be shed into the lumen of the intestine, increasing the iron loss from the body in the presence of iron overload. This scheme assigns two pools of iron in the mucosal cell—divalent iron, which is concerned with transport, and trivalent ferritin iron, which is concerned with the temporary storage of iron. Some of the latter may be eventually changed to divalent iron and transferred out of the cell, but most remains within the cell and is eventually lost into the lumen when the cell is shed from the tip of the villus (17).

Ammonium ion appears to be actively absorbed in the hamster ileum in vitro by a mechanism influenced by CO_2 (106). Urea, while not an electrolyte, is absorbed from the gut. Lifson and Hakim found that it moved by bulk flow and diffusion, the former through pores with a radius of 10 to 15 Å. (66,96).

THE CONTROL OF SALT AND WATER ABSORPTION

Some factors influencing control have already been considered. Hormonal effects on sodium and water absorption have been demonstrated, but their role under normal circumstances remains problematic. Gastrin and gastrin pentapeptide reduced the rate of absorption of sodium and water from the ileum in vitro and in dogs with Thiry-Vella loops (55,60). Obstruction of the vena cava above the level of the hepatic veins led to a decrease in the output of sodium in the feces in dogs, which was corrected by bilateral adrenalectomy. Levitan found that aldosterone increased absorption of sodium from the human colon but had no effect on the small intestine (93,94). Similarly, 2 mg of aldosterone had no effect on the water and electrolyte content of human ileostomy fluid (95).

Dietary restriction of sodium in dogs resulted in a reduction in the concentration of sodium in ileal contents (48). The Tidballs found some evidence for involvement of the vagus in the absorption of sodium chloride, since after vagotomy the reduction of absorption after atropine did not occur (144).

As with other intestinal functions, blood flow must be considered as a factor in the absorption of water and electrolyte. Hanson and Johnson demonstrated an autoregulatory control mechanism in the colon, but it appeared to be exerted through the veins rather than the large arteries (67). Unless flow is markedly reduced, it has yet to be shown that it is rate-limiting for absorption. During defecation Geber found that colonic blood flow fell 30 per cent in anesthetized dogs (57).

ABSORPTION OF WATER AND ELECTROLYTES IN MAN

Salt and water are absorbed in the proximal small intestine in man probably largely in response to osmotic gradients. In the ileum, chloride may be absorbed by a mechanism involving the secretion of bicarbonate. Potassium also may be secreted in the ileum and colon. Adrenocortical secretion may exert an influence on the absorption of sodium and water in the colon. There may be an adaptive response to a low-sodium diet.

Calcium and iron are absorbed from the proximal small intestine probably by a carrier-mediated process. Normal parathyroid function and vitamin D are necessary for normal calcium absorption. The absorption of iron is controlled in some fashion involving the relationship between iron in the absorptive cell and total body iron stores.

PATHOPHYSIOLOGY

There are a number of diseases characterized by watery diarrhea and the passage of large volumes of water and electrolytes in the stool. The underlying disturbance may be a failure of lumen-to-blood flux, excessive blood-to-lumen movement, or both. Cholera seems to be an example of the latter while the semiformed stool of the patient with an ileostomy is an example of the former. Loss of distal small intestinal content can be expected to produce deficits in body potassium and bicarbonate.

There are also examples of excessive absorption of electrolytes. In the granulomatous disease sarcoidosis there may be hypercalcemia due to increased absorption of calcium as a result of increased sensitivity to vitamin D. At one time cancer of the bladder was treated by transplanting the ureters to the sigmoid colon and excising the bladder. Some of these patients developed hyperchloremic acidosis as a result of absorption of chloride from urine.

Endocrine disorders may involve water and electrolyte absorption in the intestine. The intestinal contents in hyperaldosteronism show an increase in potassium concentration and a decrease in sodium. Water retention follows sodium retention whether the hyperaldosteronism is secondary to changes in renal blood flow or the consequence of an aldosterone-producing tumor. Certain islet-cell tumors of the pancreas produce watery diarrhea and hypokalemia, thought to be the result of secretion of polypeptide hormone by the tumor. Villous adenomas of the colon may cause hypokalemia as a result of hypersecretion.

The Absorption of Carbohydrates

The absorption of sugars from the intestine in vitro can occur against a concentration gradient and requires metabolic energy (26). The structural requirements of sugar molecules for active transport include stereospecific configurations. The process becomes saturated at higher concentrations and actively transported sugars compete with one another when present in the mucosal solution. The most likely explanation for this phenomenon is a carrier-mediated transport. (27). Active transport of sugar is inhibited by phlorizin as well as more general metabolic inhibitors. Michaelis-Menten kinetics can be demonstrated by a Lineweaver-Burk plot of the rate of absorption vs. the concentration of the sugar, as discussed earlier. Increases in the potential difference across the mucosa occur coincident with the absorption of actively transported sugars (28).

The absorption of glucose is accelerated in the presence of sodium. Ouabain (28) and certain glucosides (44) inhibit glucose transport. Sodium is also necessary for the activation of sucrase in the brush border (136). Crane proposed that sugars and sodium shared specific sites on the same carrier, as shown in Figure 9-10. In the absence of sodium, the carrier might become less efficient in transporting sugar.

On the basis of autoradiographs and the behavior of brush border preparations, Crane concluded that the entry mechanism for sugars into the surface epithelial cells was concentrated at the brush border (28). Accumulation of sugar within the cell is dependent apparently upon a continuously maintained outward sodium gradient. The unique feature of the intestinal epithelial cell lies in the fact that sodium extrusion is directed toward specific cell borders rather than across the cell membrane in general, as in most cells.

Taylor et al. found that actively transported sugars increased the rate of active absorption of sodium regardless of the extent to which the sugars were metabolized by the tissue (143). Some amino acids inhibit the transport of certain sugars, possibly by competing for the same carrier (69).

In vivo, absorption of carbohydrate proceeds rapidly. It is difficult to give sufficient glucose into the stomach to exceed the intestine's capacity for absorption (123). Glucose feeding for six weeks in rats increased the absorption and transport of glucose in the ileum (110).

In man, after a mixed meal containing glucose in a concentration of about 900 mM/L, the glucose concentration at the ligament of Treitz was about 200 mM. In the jejunum it was about 170, and in the ileum about 75 mM (13). The absorption of glucose was essentially completed in the first 50 to 100 cm of jejunum. Nearly twice as much glucose was absorbed from loops of jejunum as from loops of ileum of equal length (53).

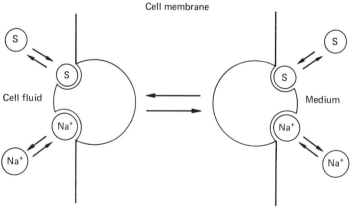

FIGURE 9-10.   Model of mobile carrier with two sites, one specific for substrates and one specific for Na. (From R. K. Crane. *Fed. Proc.* **24:** 1001, 1965.)

Holdsworth and Dawson found that the absorption of glucose was related to the load of glucose rather than the rate of perfusion of the solution or its concentration (Figure 9-11) (71). Comparison of the absorption of glucose, galactose, and fructose in man showed that similar relationships held for glucose and galactose, but fructose absorption was linearly related to the concentration of the sugar in the perfusate, as shown in Figure 9-12. This has been interpreted as evidence for absorption of fructose by facilitated diffusion rather than active transport (37).

At concentrations above 0.1 per cent glucose, sodium lack did not seem to influence glucose absorption in man, and absorption from hypotonic solutions did not increase. Assuming that the concentration of glucose in the lumen after a meal ranged from 6 to 35 mM/L, Olsen and Inglefinger concluded that most absorption of glucose in man occurred in the presence of a downhill concentration gradient. Active transport may be less important in man (111).

Absorption of glucose from the colon in man was found to be insignificant (98). Some CO_2 produced by bacterial oxidation from glucose was absorbed. Rectal administration of glucose solutions would seem to be of little value.

When the human intestine was perfused with sucrose, glucose and fructose appear in the lumen, although little or no sucrase activity could be detected in the fluid (63). This is in keeping with Crane's model of the epithelial cell in which the disaccharidases of the brush border lie on the luminal side of the barrier crossed by monosaccharides in the process of active transport. Hydrolysis may occur more rapidly than absorption. Maltose was hydrolyzed more rapidly than lactose, but the step was not rate-limiting for absorption except in lactase-deficient individuals (102).

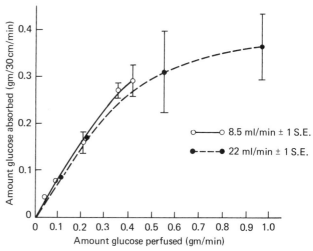

FIGURE 9-11   Absorption of glucose is related to load rather than to flow rate or concentration of test solution. (From C. D. Holdsworth and A. M. Dawson. *Clin. Sci.* **27:** 373–376, 1964.)

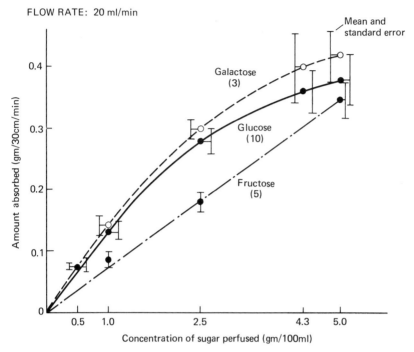

FLOW RATE: 20 ml/min

FIGURE 9-12. Absorption of glucose, galactose, and fructose in normal-subjects. Figures in brackets indicate number of subjects in each group. (From C. D. Holdsworth and A. M. Dawson. *Clin. Sci.* **27**: 373–376, 1964.)

There is little or no glucose in fasting intestinal content, so that intestinal mucosa forms an effective barrier to the transport of glucose from blood to intestinal lumen (53).

Control of intestinal absorption of sugars by nervous or hormonal mechanisms has yet to be shown under normal circumstances. Diabetes in animals and man results in increased absorption of glucose (6,147). Flores and Schedl suggested that this was due to increased uptake in the tissues, but the mechanism is unknown. Although absorption of sugar may be rapid in patients with hyperthyroidism, intestinal segments from hyperthyroid rats showed no significant change in the transfer system for hexoses (88).

The relationship between motor activity and absorption of sugar may be of significance. Parasympathomimetic drugs increased glucose absorption from intestinal loops in man, but atropine, an anticholinergic, increased the absorption of D-xylose (31,53).

ABSORPTION OF SUGARS IN MAN

Disaccharides are hydrolyzed to monosaccharides by brush-border disaccharidases in the small intestine. At some point deeper in the cell surface, hexoses enter the mucosal epithelial cell, probably under circumstances of a downhill concentration gradient after a meal. Absorption of glucose is completed in the proximal jejunum. Hormonal and nervous control mechanisms have not been shown to be of significance under normal circumstances.

PATHOPHYSIOLOGY

Impairment of the absorption of sugar in man occurs under two circumstances—deficiency of the brush-border digestive enzymes and reduction of the area of the absorptive surface. Large numbers of selected populations have been shown to lack or have significantly reduced lactase activity in specimens of small intestinal mucosa. This leads to increased amounts of lactose in the gut after drinking milk and a symptom complex including abdominal distress and diarrhea. The lactase deficiency is probably a genetic defect rather than a failure of induction in infancy. Lactase deficiency may be secondary to disease of the intestinal mucosa such as enteritis. In these patients, the blood sugar fails to rise after a meal of lactose.

Extensive resection of the small bowel, inflammatory disease of the gut, and villous atrophy as seen in adult celiac disease may be associated with impaired absorption of glucose. This may result from reduction of the absorptive surface. Malabsorption of a nonmetabolized sugar such as D-xylose may be detected by measuring the urinary excretion of the sugar after a test meal. The blood levels after a glucose meal are too variable in normal subjects to provide a satisfactory test for malabsorption.

Absorption of Proteins, Peptides, and Amino Acids

Except for the first days of life, absorption of intact proteins from the intestine does not normally occur. In some animals, particularly ruminants, immunoglobulins are absorbed during the first days of life by a process of pinocytosis (105). The Golgi apparatus may show changes during absorption (1). The termination of absorption of these proteins can be hastened by cortisol or delayed by starvation. In primates absorption of antibodies has been reported in the neonatal period. In adults the normal daily fecal loss of protein is 3 to 15 gm (107). Since this represents less than 10 per cent of the total amount of protein entering the gut from dietary sources and endogenous secretions, most of the protein is digested and absorbed. Absorption of insulin has been reported when the digestive activity of the intestine was inhibited.

Similarly, with the exception of small quantities of glycyl-glycine, no peptides have been found to be transported from the mucosal to the serosal side of gut segments in vitro. Most proteins and peptides are absorbed only after they have been hydrolyzed to their constituent amino acids (103). As in the case of the disaccharidases, peptidases have been located in the brush border of the intestinal epithelium. Amino acids appear in the mucosal solution after exposure to dipeptides, suggesting, as with sugars, that the peptidases lie more superficially than the barrier crossed by transport into the cell (*103*). Fisher thought that if peptides were absorbed they would be more likely to appear in the lymphatics than in the portal blood (*49*).

The absorption of amino acids bears many similarities to that of sugars. An energy-dependent active transport process has been demonstrated for certain amino acids, particularly those of the L form (*158*). A carrier-mediated mechanism is suspected. Saturation of the mechanism can be shown. Figure 9-13 shows a Lineweaver-Burk plot for the absorption of amino acids in the everted hamster gut sac. Competition can be shown between amino acids.

On the basis of these factors, at least four separate mechanisms exist for the transport of the following groups of amino acids: neutral amino acids, basic amino acids, dicarboxylic amino acids, and the group of imino acids and proline (*127*). Using gut segments, the absorption of L-selenomethionine was greatest in segments from the second quarter of the hamster intestine (*101*). McLeod and Tyor found that three basic amino acids were transported maximally in the distal hamster intestine (*100*).

Replacement of sodium in the bathing solution of everted intestinal sacs

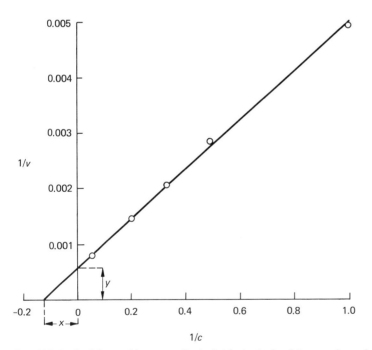

FIGURE 9-13.   Lineweaver-Burk plot for L-alanine $1/c$ = reciprocal of amino-acid concentration (mM) $1/v$ = reciprocal of corresponding transport rate (μmoles/gm. dry wt./hr.). (From D. M. Matthews, and L. Laster. *Gut* **6**: 411–426, 1965: Reproduced by permission of the Authors and Editor.)

reduced valine transport, and replacement of chloride with sulfate reduced valine uptake (124). Ouabain reduced amino acid transport with little effect on hexoses (108). The effect was more pronounced in the absence of potassium.

Curran suggested that the transport of amino acids utilized the energy of the sodium extrusion mechanism and therefore constituted a special form of "active transport" (32). There is also evidence for competition between amino acids and glucose for transport. Fructose had no effect (4).

In man, perfusion studies showed retardation of absorption of individual amino acids from mixtures when the concentrations reached 3 mM. Absorption was fastest for methionine and slowest for threonine in the mixtures (2). Like glucose, the absorption of protein given as albumin was complete in the first 50 to 100 cm of jejunum (13). Schedl et al. found that L-methionine was absorbed more rapidly in the proximal small intestine. Using Lineweaver-Burk plots, they showed that the concentration of methionine at which absorption was half-maximal (K_t) was three times greater in the proximal than in the distal gut (133). This suggested that different transport mechanisms were involved.

Other evidence for separate mechanisms comes from the differences between intestinal transport of cystine and cysteine. Both are transported by active processes, but only cysteine can be recovered within cells. In the disease cystinuria, cysteine uptake is normal but the uptake of cystine is defective (126).

As with sugars, little is known of the factors controlling the absorption of amino acids. Semistarvation increased the absorption of amino acids (83). Thyroid hormone decreased the absorption of valine, while thyroparathyroidectomy increased it in everted gut sacs from rats. Parathyroidectomy alone had no effect (76). Cummins and Almy reported that cholinergic drugs increased the motility of intestinal loops in man and increased the absorption of methionine (31). Exclusion of bile and pancreatic juice had no effect on the absorption of amino acids (158).

ABSORPTION OF AMINO ACIDS IN MAN

Absorption of amino acids is essentially complete in the first 100 cm of jejunum (13). Like glucose, the sodium requirements for the absorption of glycine and alanine are low (49a). However the kinetics of absorption suggest that these two amino acids share a common active mechanism for transport. Peptidases in the brush border are responsible for the hydrolysis of peptides in the intestinal content and lie more superficially than the site of active transport. Little is known of nervous or hormonal control systems.

PATHOPHYSIOLOGY

Increased amounts of protein in the feces usually indicate excessive protein loss either in the form of inflammatory exudate as in colitis or as leaking into the gut from the blood. The latter phenomenon, known as protein-losing enteropathy, may occur in constrictive pericarditis or lymphatic obstruction. It may be quantitated by measuring the appearance of labeled chromium in the feces after giving chromium-labeled albumin intravenously.

A number of defects in the transport of specific amino acids across the intestine have been identified and presumed to represent genetically determined defects. In some instances, a transport defect exists in both the small intestine and the renal tubule (126). The defect may represent an enzyme catalyzing a change in the amino acid during its transport or a defective carrier protein.

The Absorption of Fat

The mechanism by which fat in the form of micelles enters the mucosal epithelial cells and later leaves as triglyceride is unknown. The uptake of micellar fatty acids and monoglycerides is independent of temperature and does not require energy (80). Much effort has been expended to find a structural basis for fat absorption, using electron microscopy. As a result of the appearance of fat droplets following feeding of triglycerides, early investigators suggested that fat might enter epithelial cells by the process of pinocytosis. Current work fails to support this concept (141). Autoradiographs indicated that fat entered the cells as fatty acids at zero-degree temperature but was converted to triglyceride at body temperature. Biochemical and morphologic observations seem to agree that in some unknown fashion the fatty acids and monoglycerides leave the micelles and enter the absorptive cell, while the bile salt and phospholipid remain in the lumen of the intestine. Hogben vigorously supported the concept that fatty acids entered cells by diffusion (70).

The second phase of absorption concerns the reesterification of fatty acids and monoglycerides to triglycerides (77,78,138). This could occur by complete hydrolysis to fatty acids and resynthesis via a glycerophosphate pathway or by acylation of the monoglyceride. The enzymes responsible for both pathways were localized to the microsomal fraction of mucosal cells in cat intestine and to the rough-surface vesicle fractions (15). Senior and Isselbacher demonstrated an intracellular monoglyceride lipase which could hydrolyze monoglyceride to free fatty acids and glycerol (137).

The source of the glycerol in resynthesis of triglycerides is of interest. Although earlier work suggested that dietary free glycerol was not incorporated into triglyceride within the mucosa, more recent studies report that as much as 30 per cent of labeled glycerol in the intestine could be recovered in triglycerides from the thoracic duct (80).

The final stage in the absorption of long-chain fatty acids is the formation of chylomicrons. The triglycerides are surrounded by an outer coating of phospholipid and cholesterol. This process, too, occurs in the microsomes (79).

The microscopic appearance of the fat droplet surrounded by a membrane within the cell suggested that the membrane might be derived from the endoplasmic reticulum. The rough endoplasmic reticulum is probably involved in the synthesis of chylomicron protein. Figure 9-14 shows the process of absorption of long-chain fatty acids and, for comparison, the absorption of medium-chain (8 to 10 carbon atoms) fatty acids. The latter are not reesterified and pass directly into the portal vein. Under normal circumstances, medium-chain-length triglycerides are hydrolyzed to fatty acids by pancreatic lipase and absorbed as fatty acids. However, in the absence of pancreatic secretion, significant amounts of MCT are absorbed as triglycerides and then hydrolyzed within the mucosal cell (120,128). When long-chain triglycerides were given with MCT, small amounts of the MCT appeared in the lymph as triglyceride (85).

Do endogenous fatty acids contribute to chylomicron triglyceride during absorption of fat? Reeve and Franks found no stimulating effect of feeding LCT on endogenous fatty acid synthesis and suggested that synthesis of fatty acids occurred by elongation of preexisting fatty acids (122). The membrane of chylomicrons can be isolated as "ghosts" and was found to consist of a mosaic of small amounts of protein, free cholesterol, and a monolayer of phospholipid (160).

The capacity of the intestine to absorb fat is more limited than that for carbohydrate and protein. It was possible to exceed the capacity of ileal loops in dogs to absorb fat, and in rats duodenal infusions of emulsified fats showed that the maximal absorptive capacity for triolein was about 300 μM/hr, while for trioctanoin, a medium-chain-length triglyceride, it was nearly 1,600 (4,20).

Studies using labeled fat in man show that the 2-monoglyceride pathway was the major route for the resynthesis of triglyceride within the intestinal

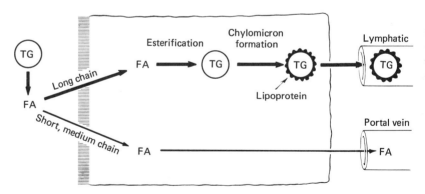

FIGURE 9-14. Pathways of lipid transport in the mucosa and step where inhibition of protein synthesis interferes with fat absorption. (From K. J. Isselbacher.: Mechanisms of absorption of long and medium chain triglycerides. In: *Medium Chain Triglycerides.* Edited by J. R. Senior. Philadelphia: University of Pennsylvania Press, 1968, pp. 21–38.)

mucosa (81). Little dietary free glycerol appeared in lymph. Holt studied a patient with chyluria and concluded that glycerol released in the intestinal lumen during triglyceride hydrolysis may be reutilized for glyceride synthesis in the mucosa (72).

CONTROL OF FAT ABSORPTION

As with the other dietary constituents, there is little evidence of significant neuroendocrine control of fat absorption. Adrenalectomized rats showed a mild malabsorption of fat and a deficiency of the activities of enzymes concerned with the resynthesis of triglycerides (125). Hypophysectomy increased esterification of myristic acid in gut slices in rats, while cortisone and L-thyroxine reduced it (58).

THE ABSORPTION OF FAT IN MAN

Monoglycerides in micellar form bind to the intestinal mucosa by a passive, nonenergy-dependent process. In some unknown fashion, possibly diffusion, monoglycerides enter the mucosal cells. The remainder of the micelle returns to the intestinal lumen. In normal man, this process is completed in the upper jejunum (13). Once inside the cell, the monoglyceride is reesterified to triglyceride by enzyme systems in the microsomes. The newly formed triglyceride is surrounded by an envelope of protein, phospholipid, and cholesterol and discharged into the lymphatics as chylomicrons. The source of the glycerol for reesterification and the details of chylomicron synthesis are unknown. This course of events applies to the usual dietary triglycerides containing 16 to 18 carbon atoms in their fatty acids (long-chain fatty acids or LCT). Medium-chain-length triglycerides (8 to 10 carbon atoms, MCT) are hydrolyzed to fatty acids in the lumen and traverse the mucosal cells without reesterification. They enter the portal vein rather than the lymphatics.

PATHOPHYSIOLOGY

In the majority of malabsorption syndromes, it is the excessive excretion of fat in the stools (steatorrhea) that provides the best quantitative measure of the absorptive defect as well as determining the gross appearance of the stool and the patient's description of it. The amount of fat in the stools over a three-day period, provided that the patient is receiving at least 70 gm of fat per day in his diet, is the standard quantitative assay of malabsorption. Such a procedure does not distinguish between failure of digestion, as in insufficient secretion of pancreatic lipase, and true malabsorption, with a reduction of absorbing surface and deranged function of the absorptive cells. Other evidence of pancreatic insufficiency and the appearance of the small bowel on biopsy usually suffice to differentiate the two. The interesting disease abetalipoproteinemia may provide an example of a disturbance in chylomicron formation. Fat accumulates within the mucosal cells in this disease and there are no beta-lipoproteins in the plasma. Medium-chain-length triglycerides should offer a means of bypassing the defect and, indeed, increased absorption of fat has been reported in patients with the syndrome given MCT. Similarly in other malabsorptive diseases, MCT is absorbed better than LCT. However, it remains to be seen whether anything other than a source of calories for the liver has been accomplished. This itself may be very important for patients with only short segments of intestine remaining after surgical resections.

The Absorption of Cholesterol

The absorption of the group of substances including a sterol nucleus is worthy of study because of their unique role in metabolism and their possible significance in the genesis of atherosclerosis. The incorporation of cholesterol into micelles with bile salts, phospholipid, and monoglycerides has already been described. One of the features of this complex is that hydrolysis of cholesterol esters to free cholesterol is accelerated fourfold (145). Pancreatic secretion contains an enzyme, cholesterol hydrolase, which produces much more complete hydrolysis of cholesterol esters in a micellar solution. Bile salts may function as cofactors for cholesterol esterase as well as acting as surface-active agents. Mucoprotein on the surface of epithelial cells has the property of binding cholesterol but is probably not involved in the transfer into the cell. The mechanism of penetration of cholesterol into the cell is unknown.

Within the cell, cholesterol mixes with a small pool of free cholesterol. Esterification occurs as one of the processes involved in the formation of chylomicrons; the latter are composed of approximately 80 per cent ester and 20 per cent free cholesterol. The cellular cholesterol esterase lies deep to the brush border and was found to be present in the cell supernatant in largest percentage. Pancreatic cholesterol esterase increases the activity of mucosal esterase. The fatty acids used in esterification reflect the composition of the fatty acid pool, including both dietary and endogenous fatty acids. There is some evidence that oleic acid may be preferentially esterified with cholesterol (Fig. 9-15).

The formation of chylomicrons is poorly understood. Inhibitors of protein synthesis such as puromycin interfere with chylomicron formation without affecting mucosal glyceride synthesis (Fig. 9-14). This is compatible with an inability of the ribosomes to synthesize protein. Chylomicrons may be produced in the endoplasmic reticulum. Cholesterol is transported exclusively in the lymphatics from the intestine.

Other sterols inhibit the absorption of cholesterol. The absorptive mechanism is presumably similar. Schedl and Clifton found no evidence of an active-transport process for cortisol in man (132).

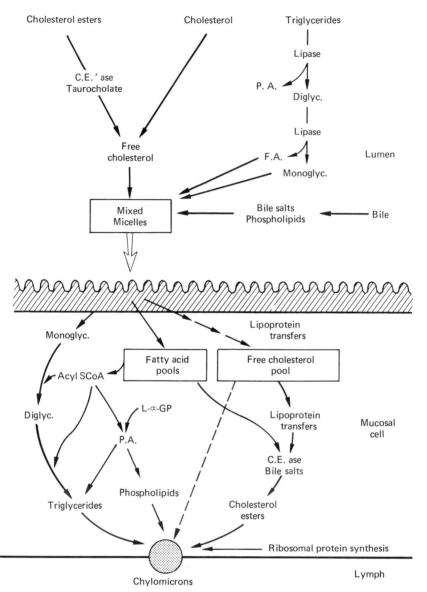

FIGURE   9-15.   Mechanism of cholesterol absorption. Abbreviations: C. E.[1] ase, cholesterol esterase; F. A., fatty acids; Diglyc.: diglycerides; Monoglyc., monoglycerides; L-α-GP, L-α-glycerolphosphate; P. A., phosphatidic acid. (From C. R. Treadwell, and G. V. Vahouny. Cholesterol absorption. In: *Handbook of Physiology*. Section 6: Alimentary Tract, Vol. 3: Absorption. Edited by C. F. Code. Washington, D.C. American Physiological Society, 1968, pp. 1402–1438.)

THE CONTROL OF CHOLESTEROL SYNTHESIS

Recent developments assign an important role to the intestine in cholesterol synthesis. Cholesterol synthesis in the liver is related to the amount of cholesterol in the diet, increasing with lower amounts of dietary cholesterol. In squirrel monkeys on a low-cholesterol diet, the liver and ileum were the most active sites of cholesterologenesis, followed in order by the colon, esophagus, and proximal small intestine. Under normal circumstances Wilson found that 1.5 to 2.0 mg of cholesterol synthesized in the monkey's intestinal wall reached the circulation each day (154).

Following feeding of cholesterol, there was a marked suppression of hepatic cholesterologenesis with little change in intestinal production. However, diversion of bile salts from the intestine for 48 hours increased small intestinal cholesterol synthesis six- to eight-fold, while only increasing hepatic synthesis by a factor of two. These results indicate an important control mechanism for the synthesis of cholesterol in the intestine. The cells appear to respond to the level of bile salts in the intestine, increasing cholesterol synthesis when bile salts were diverted or when absorption was prevented by the administration of a binding resin cholestyramine (43).

The Absorption of Bile Salts

The enterohepatic circulation of bile salts has already been mentioned. An exciting recent development has been the characterization of a specific transport system in the ileum for their absorption (149). Normally only a small fraction of bile salts escape reabsorption. They are returned almost quantitatively to the liver via the portal vein, being carried bound to plasma proteins. Bile salts in the feces are entirely unconjugated and exhibit a number of modifications in structure due to bacterial action. In guinea pigs with ligated intestinal loops, 15 mg of taurocholate injected into the ileum was recovered almost quantitatively in the bile. The taurocholate appeared about an hour later than after intravenous administration. Lack and Weiner used everted gut sac preparations to demonstrate an active-transport mechanism for bile salts in the ileum but not in the proximal small intestine (68). It was inhibited by metabolic poisons and sensitive to the presence of sodium. Saturation of the system occurred with higher levels of bile salt. Competitive inhibition between bile salts was shown in the guinea pig (68) and rat (73).

In man Borgstrom et al. found that labeled bile salts appeared in duodenal content more rapidly when injected into the ileum (14). Subsequent studies showed that bile salts exerted their role in the absorption of fat in the proximal intestine but were reabsorbed in the ileum. Bile salts can be absorbed by diffusion and nonionic diffusion elsewhere in the small intestine.

Malabsorption of bile salts due to disease or absence of the ileum might be expected to lead to malabsorption of fat (7). Bacterial overgrowth in the small intestine may alter the structure of bile salts so that absorption cannot occur by an active process. In the latter group, antibiotics might be of help at least temporarily. The possibility that deconjugated bile salts may exert a toxic effect on intestinal epithelial cells remains to be demonstrated in man.

Absorption of Vitamins

The importance of vitamins in nutrition warrants special consideration for their absorption (104). The fat-soluble vitamins would be expected to follow pathways similar to that of lipids. Goodman et al. found that vitamin A of dietary origin was almost completely esterified with long-chain fatty acids which were then transported in the lymph in association with chylomicrons (62). The intestinal mucosa cleaves carotene into two molecules of retinal. In man there is a limited ability to absorb carotene unchanged.

The water-soluble vitamins, with the exception of vitamin B_{12}, have been of little interest to students of absorption. Folic acid is absorbed largely from the upper small intestine and may have to be in a conjugated form for absorption. The maximum absorptive capacity for thiamine in man is said to be only a few milligrams. Present evidence would suggest that the absorption of ascorbic acid and riboflavin is by passive diffusion.

The absorption of vitamin B_{12} involves the formation of a complex of the vitamin with intrinsic factor secreted by the stomach. Intrinsic factor is a polypeptide of undetermined structure. Other factors will bind vitamin B_{12} but do not participate in the absorptive mechanism (18). Studies with everted gut sacs showed that the transport system was localized in the ileum (156). Cooper found that intestinal scrapings from the ileum of normal subjects, after feeding labeled B_{12}, contained the vitamin bound to intrinsic factor. Donaldson et al. reported that the brush border of ileal mucosa from hamsters took up vitamin B_{12} in the presence of intrinsic factor. Brush borders from the jejunum did not show this property. Uptake was much reduced in the absence of divalent cations, and the process did not require energy (45). Wilson suggested that absorption occurred by the process of pinocytosis (156). In vivo studies by one group of investigators failed to demonstrate the specificity of transport in the ileum (56).

Lack of production of intrinsic factor by the stomach leads to malabsorption of B_{12} and the disease pernicious anemia. Stores of B_{12} in the liver may delay the development of the disease for as long as seven years after total gastric resection. Disease of the terminal ileum such as enteritis may also produce an anemia similar to pernicious anemia. Surgical removal or bypass of the ileum will have similar effects. Bacterial overgrowth in blind loops may also interfere with absorption of B_{12}.

The absorption of B_{12} may be used as a semiquantitative test of absorption. After loading the patient with intramuscular B_{12}, radioactive B_{12} is given by mouth and the urinary excretion of radioactivity followed. Failure of less than 5 per cent of the radioactivity to appear in the urine indicates malabsorption. Repeating the test in the presence of intrinsic factor makes it possible to specifically indicate deficiency of intrinsic factor as the cause of malabsorption if absorption returns to normal. Interpretation is complicated by the variability of results on repeated tests, particularly in the lower range of normal.

Absorption from the Gallbladder

The composition of human hepatic bile has been given in Table 6-1. Admirand and Small found bile salt concentrations in human normal gallbladder bile of 135 ± 65 mM/L, compared to 40–160 in Table 6-1 (3). Bicarbonate concentrations fall, chloride concentrations fall, while the concentrations of sodium and potassium rise. The bile remains isotonic but the pH falls into the range just below 7. The mechanism by which these changes are brought about is under extensive investigation. Diamond devised a preparation of the gallbladder in vitro which permitted the collection of fluid moving from mucosa to serosa in an atmosphere of moist oxygen (36). He found that the osmolarity of the transported fluid bore a direct relationship to that of the mucosal fluid over a wide range. Wheeler used a similar preparation and found that net water flux was proportional to solute transport. Isethionate could be substituted for chloride in the mucosal solution if sodium were the cation, but not if choline was substituted for sodium (150). Experiments with an everted gallbladder in vitro confirmed the importance of sodium (117). As a result of these experiments, the concept of a neutral coupled sodium chloride pump has been suggested as the concentrating mechanism (39,40, 151,152). The observations were confirmed in vivo (151). The nonspecificity of the anion requirement was shown by Whitlock and Wheeler, who found that bicarbonate, lactate, and proprionate could substitute for chloride (152). The divalent ion sulfate was not transported. Dietschy found that if bile salts were substituted for chloride, an additional fraction of water was absorbed, presumably because the bile salts produced a degree of hypotonicity in the mucosal solution (40).

The potential difference across the gallbladder wall is very small under normal circumstances: 0.8 ± 0.6 (39). However, it can be shown to vary in vivo with the concentration of sodium. The distribution of potassium concentrations can be predicted from the Nernst equation, suggesting that potassium moves in response to diffusion potentials (41).

The transport of water has been studied in the in vitro preparation. In gallbladders transporting water, the lateral intercellular spaces were dilated. Without transport, there was no distention. When sodium or chloride were omitted from the mucosal solution, distention did not occur. Sodium was present in high concentrations in the intercellular space, and an ATPase is known to be present in the lateral plasma membrane (82). Similar considerations lead to the suggestion that sodium is actively extruded into the lateral intercellular spaces, and water follows the osmotic gradient (37,38,42). The concentration of sodium would be greater at the apical end of the lateral space and would fall as the base of the cells approached. Figure 9-16 is a diagrammatic representation of the mechanism. Grim still preferred the mechanism of pinocytosis to explain water transport in the gallbladder (65).

Ballantyne and Wood found a beta-glucuronidase in the cytoplasm of epithelial cells of the mammalian gallbladder. There were significant species differences and the enzyme activity was higher in males. They suggested that it might play a role in sodium transport (8).

Ostrow described a nonenergy-dependent transport of unconjugated bilirubin in the gallbladder (113). Other investigators also observed absorption of bilirubin and found that ligating the vascular pedicle decreased absorption (59).

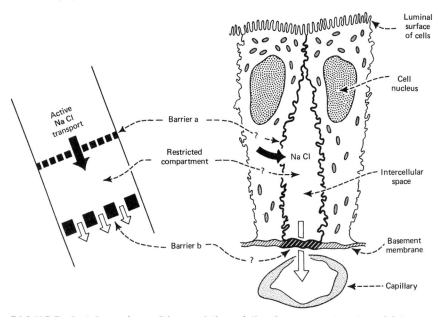

FIGURE 9-16.   A possible correlation of the three-compartment model to an-
atomical structures within the gall bladder epithelium, based on the experimental data of
Kaye et al. and Whitlock et al. (From J. M. Dietschy: *Gastroenterology* **50:** 692–707. © 1966,
The Williams & Wilkins Co., Baltimore, Md. 21202, U.S.A.)

CONTROL OF ABSORPTION BY THE GALLBLADDER

Diamond made the provocative observation that oxytocin inhibited absorption from the gallbladder in vitro while vasopressin had no effect (39). Using human gallbladders, Onstad et al. found that cholecystokinin reduced the weight of everted gallbladders and increased muscular contractions. Norepinephrine led to a gain in weight (112).

PATHOPHYSIOLOGY

Although there is little direct application of these findings to human disease, the possibility that they may lead to an understanding of the cause of gallstones is ample justification for considering them. Gallstones occur in as many as 10 per cent of the population over 55, and the cost in time and effort for removing gallbladders is an important factor in the cost of medical care. If disease of the gallbladder wall leads to a change in the composition of bile favoring the development of stones, then an understanding of the normal concentrating mechanism is the first step toward the pathogenic mechanisms in cholelithiasis.

References

1. Adamstone, F. B. Response of the Golgi apparatus of absorptive cells of the intestinal epithelium of the rat to the ingestion of protein. *Amer. J. Anat.* **103:** 437–465, 1958.
2. Adibi, S. A., and S. J. Gray. Intestinal absorption of essential amino acids in man. *Gastroenterology* **52:** 837–845, 1967.
3. Admirand, W. H., and D. M. Small. The physicochemical basis of cholesterol gallstone formation in man. *J. Clin. Invest.* **47:** 1043–1052, 1968.
4. Annegers, J. H. Absorption of lipid and cholate from ileal loops in unanesthetized dogs. *Am. J. Physiol.* **191:** 75–80, 1957.
5. Annegers, J. H. Some effects of hexoses on the absorption of amino acids. *Am. J. Physiol.* **210:** 701–704, 1966.
6. Aulsebrook, K. A. Intestinal transport of glucose and sodium: changes in alloxan diabetes and effects of insulin. *Experentia* **21:** 346–347, 1965.
7. Austad, W. I., L. Lack, and M. P. Tyor. Importance of bile acids and of an intact distal small intestine for fat absorption. *Gastroenterology* **52:** 638–646, 1967.
8. Ballantyne, B., and W. G. Wood. Biochemical and histochemical observations on β-glucuronidase in the mammalian gallbladder. *Am. J. Digest. Dis.* **13:** 551–557, 1968.
9. Barry, R. J. C. Electrical changes in relation to transport. *Brit. Med. Bull.* **23:** 266–269, 1967.
10. Bejar, J., S. A. Broitman, and N. Zamcheck. Effect of vagotomy upon the small intestine. *Gut* **9:** 87–90, 1968.
11. Benson, J. A., Jr., and A. J. Rampone. Gastrointestinal absorption. *Ann. Rev. Physiol.* **28:** 201–226, 1966.

12. Booth, C. C. Effect of location along the small intestine on absorption of nutrients. In: *Handbook of Physiology*. Section 6: Alimentary Tract. Vol. III: Absorption. Edited by C. F. Code. Washington, D.C.: American Physiological Society, 1968, pp. 1513–1528.

13. Borgstrom, B., A. Dahlquist, G. Lundh, and J. Sjovall. Studies of intestinal digestion and absorption in the human. *J. Clin. Invest.* **36:** 1521–1536, 1957.

14. Borgstrom, B., G. Lundh, and A. Hofmann. The site of absorption of conjugated bile salts in man. *Gastroenterology* **45:** 229–238, 1963.

15. Brindley, D. N., and G. Hubscher. The intracellular distribution of the enzymes catalyzing the biosynthesis of glycerides in the intestinal mucosa. *Biochim Biophys. Acta.* **106:** 495–509, 1965.

16. Cairnie, A. B., L. F. Lamerton, and G. G. Steele. Cell proliferation studies in the intestinal epithelium of the rat. *Exp. Cell Res.* **39:** 528–553, 1965.

17. Callender, S. T. Intestinal mucosa and iron absorption. *Brit. Med. Bull.* **23:** 263–265, 1967.

18. Castle, W. B. Gastric intrinsic factor and vitamin B_{12} absorption. In: *The Handbook of Physiology*. Section 6: Alimentary Tract. Vol. III: Absorption. Edited by C. F. Code. Washington, D.C.: American Physiological Society, 1968, pp. 1529–1552.

19. Clark, I. Effect of magnesium ions on calcium and phosphorus metabolism. *Am. J. Physiol.* **214:** 348–356, 1968.

20. Clark, S. B., and P. R. Holt. Rate-limiting steps in steady-state intestinal absorption of Trioctanoin-1-^{14}C: effect of biliary and pancreatic flow diversion. *J. Clin. Invest.* **47:** 612–623, 1968.

21. Clarkson, T. W., A. C. Cross, and S. R. Toole. Electrical potentials across isolated small intestine of the rat. *Am. J. Physiol.* **200:** 1233–1235, 1961.

22. Cocco, A. E., M. J. Dohrmann, and T. R. Hendrix. Reconstruction of normal jejunal biopsies: Three-dimensional histology. *Gastroenterology* **51:** 24–31, 1966.

23. Conrad, M. E., B. I. Benjamin, H. L. Williams, and A. L. Foy. Human absorption of hemoglobin-iron. *Gastroenterology* **53:** 5–10, 1967.

24. Cooper, B. A. Complex of intrinsic factor and B_{12} in human ileum during vitamin B_{12} absorption. *Am. J. Physiol.* **214:** 832–835, 1968.

25. Cooper, H., R. Levitan, J. S. Fordtran, and F. J. Inglefinger. A method for studying absorption of water and solute from human small intestine. *Gastroenterology* **50:** 1–7, 1966.

26. Crane, R. K. Intestinal absorption of sugars. *Physiol. Rev.* **40:** 789–825, 1960.

27. Crane, R. K. Hypothesis for mechanism of intestinal active transport of sugars. *Fed. Proc.* **21:** 891–895, 1962.

28. Crane, R. K. Absorption of sugars. In: *Handbook of Physiology*. Section 6: Alimentary Tract. Vol. III: Absorption. Edited by C. F. Code. Washington, D.C.: American Physiological Society, 1968, pp. 1323–1352.

29. Creamer, B. The turnover of the epithelium of the small intestine. *Brit. Med. Bull.* **23:** 226–230, 1967.

30. Crosby, W. H. Iron absorption. In: *Handbook of Physiology*. Section 6: Alimentary Tract. Vol. III: Absorption. Edited by C. F. Code. Washington, D.C.: American Physiological Society, 1968, pp. 1553–1570.

31. Cummins, A. J., and T. P. Almy. Studies on the relationship between motility and absorption in the human small intestine. *Gastroenterology* **23:** 179–190, 1953.

32. Curran, P. F. Coupling between transport processes in intestine. *Physiologist* **11**: 3–23, 1968.

33. D'Agostino, A., W. F. Leadbetter, and W. B. Schwartz. Alterations in the ionic composition of isotonic saline solution instilled into the colon. *J. Clin. Invest.* **32**: 444–448, 1953.

34. Davis, J. O., W. C. Ball, R. C. Bahn, and M. J. Goodkind. Relationship of adrenocortical and anterior pituitary function to fecal excretion of sodium and potassium. *Am. J. Physiol.* **196**: 149–152, 1959.

35. Deren, J. J. Development of intestinal structure and function. In: *Handbook of Physiology*. Section 6: Alimentary Tract. Vol. III: Absorption. Edited by C. F. Code. Washington, D.C.: American Physiological Society, 1968, pp. 1099–1124.

36. Diamond, J. M. Transport of salt and water in rabbit and guinea pig gallbladder. *J. Gen. Physiol.* **48**: 1–14, 1964.

37. Diamond, J. M. The mechanism of isotonic water transport. *J. Gen. Physiol.* **48**: 15–42, 1964.

38. Diamond, J. M., and J. McD. Tormey. Role of long extracellular channels in fluid transport across epithelia. *Nature* **210**: 817–820, 1966.

39. Diamond, J. M. The concentrating activity of the gallbladder. In: *The Biliary System*. Edited by W. Taylor. Oxford: Blackwell Scientific Publications. 1967, pp. 495–514.

40. Dietschy, J. M. Water and solute movement across the wall of the everted rabbit gallbladder. *Gastroenterology* **47**: 395–408, 1964.

41. Dietschy, M. J., and E. W. Moore. Diffusion potentials and potassium distribution across the gallbladder wall. *J. Clin. Invest.* **43**: 1551–1560, 1964.

42. Dietschy, J. M. Recent developments in solute and water transport across the gallbladder epithelium. *Gastroenterology* **50**: 692–707, 1966.

43. Dietschy, J. M., and J. D. Wilson. Cholesterol synthesis in the squirrel monkey: Relative rates of synthesis in various tissues and mechanisms of control. *J. Clin. Invest.* **47**: 166–174, 1968.

44. Despopoulos, A. Glucose transport in hamster intestine: Inhibition by glucosides. *Am. J. Physiol.* **211**: 1329–1333, 1966.

45. Donaldson, R. M., I. L. Mackenzie, and J. S. Trier. Intrinsic factor-mediated attachment of vitamin B_{12} to brush borders and microvillous membranes of hamster intestine. *J. Clin. Invest.* **46**: 1215–1228, 1967.

46. Dowling, R. H. Sites of absorption. In: *Postgraduate Gastroenterology*. Edited by T. J. Thomson and I. E. Gillespie. London: Bailliere, Tindall and Cassell, 1966, pp. 22–29.

47. Dowling, R. H. Compensatory changes in intestinal absorption. *Brit. Med. Bull.* **23**: 275–278, 1967.

48. Field, H., Jr., R. E. Dailey, R. S. Boyd, and L. Swell. Effect of restriction of dietary sodium on electrolyte composition of the contents of the terminal ileum. *Am. J. Physiol.* **179**: 477–480, 1954.

49. Fisher, R. B. Absorption of proteins. *Brit. Med. Bull.* **23**: 241–246, 1967.

49a. Fleshler, B., J. H. Butt, and J. D. Wismar. Absorption of glycine and L-alanine by the human jejunum. *J. Clin. Invest.* **45**: 1433–1441, 1966.

50. Flores, P., and H. P. Schedl. Intestinal transport of 3-*O-methyl*-D-glucose in the normal and alloxan-diabetic rat. *Am. J. Physiol.* **214**: 725–729, 1968.

51. Fordtran, J. S., F. C. Rector, Jr., M. F. Ewton, N. Soter, and J. Kinney. Permeability characteristics of the human small intestine. *J. Clin. Invest.* **44:** 1935–1944, 1965.

52. Fordtran, J. S., F. C. Rector, Jr., and N. W. Carter. The mechanisms of sodium absorption in human small intestine. *J. Clin. Invest.* **47:** 884–900, 1968.

53. Fordtran, J. S., and F. J. Inglefinger. Absorption of water, electrolytes and sugars from the human gut. In: *Handbook of Physiology.* Section 6: Alimentary Tract. Vol. III: Absorption. Edited by C. F. Code. Washington D.C.: American Physiological Society, 1968, pp. 1457–1490.

54. French, A. B., I. F. Brown, C. J. Good, and G. M. McLeod. Comparison of pheonol red and polyethyleneglycol as nonabsorbable markers for the study of intestinal absorption in humans. *Am. J. Dig. Dis.* **13:** 558–564, 1968.

55. Gardner, J. S., G. W. Peskin, J. J. Cerda, and F. P. Brooks. Alterations of in vitro fluid and electrolyte absorption by gastrointestinal hormones. *Am. J. Surg.* **113:** 57–64, 1967.

56. Gazet, J. C., and I. McColl. Absorption of B_{12} from the small intestine. Study in man, monkey, cat and dog. *Brit. J. Surg.* **54:** 128–131, 1967.

57. Geber, W. F. Functional hemodynamics of the colon. *Angiology* **15:** 366–370, 1964.

58. Gelb, A. M. The effect of hypophysectomy on esterification of fatty acids by the small intestine in vitro. *Clin. Res.* **12:** 447, 1964.

59. Gerolami, A., and H. Sarles. Etude de l'absorption des Sels biliares par La Vesicule de Chat in situ. *Rev. Franc. Etud. Clin. Biol.* **13:** 172–175, 1968.

60. Gingell, J. C., M. W. Davies, and R. Shields. Effect of a synthetic gastrin-like pentapeptide upon intestinal transport of sodium potassium and water. *Gut* **9:** 111–116, 1968.

61. Goldschmidt, S. On the mechanism of absorption from the intestine. *Physiol. Rev.* **1:** 421–453, 1921.

62. Goodman, D. S., R. Blomstrand, B. Werner, H. S. Huang, and T. Shiratori. The intestinal absorption and metabolism of vitamin A and carotene in man. *J. Clin. Invest.* **45:** 1615–1623, 1966.

63. Gray, G. M., and F. J. Inglefinger. Intestinal absorption of sucrose in man: Interrelation of hydrolysis and monosaccharide product absorption. *J. Clin. Invest.* **45:** 388–398, 1966.

64. Greenberger, N. J., and R. D. Ruppert. Inhibition of protein synthesis: A mechanism for the production of impaired iron absorption. *Science* **153:** 315–316, 1966.

65. Grim, E. A mechanism for absorption of sodium chloride solutions from the canine gallbladder. *Am. J. Physiol.* **205:** 247–254, 1963.

66. Hakim, A. A., and N. Lifson. Urea transport across dog intestinal mucosa in vitro. *Am. J. Physiol.* **206:** 1315–1320, 1964.

67. Hanson, K. M., and P. C. Johnson. Pressure-flow relationships in isolated dog colon. *Am. J. Physiol.* **212:** 574–578, 1967.

68. Heaton, K. W., and L. Lack. Ileal bile salt transport: Mutual inhibition in an in vivo system. *Am. J. Physiol.* **214:** 585–590, 1968.

69. Hindmarsh, J. T., D. Kilby, and G. Wiseman. Effect of amino acids on sugar absorption. *J. Physiol.* **186:** 166–174, 1966.

70. Hogben, C. A. M. Fat absorption: A transport problem. *Gastroenterology* **50:** 51–55, 1966.

71. Holdsworth, C. D., and A. M. Dawson. The absorption of monosaccharides in man. *Clin. Sci.* **27**: 371–379, 1964.

72. Holt, P. R. Utilization of glycerol-C^{14} for intestinal glyceride esterification: studies in a patient with chyluria. *J. Clin. Invest.* **43**: 349–356, 1964.

73. Holt, P. R. Competitive inhibition of intestinal bile salt absorption in the rat. *Am. J. Physiol.* **210**: 635–639, 1966.

74. Hubel, K. A. Bicarbonate secretion in rat ileum and its dependence on intraluminal chloride. *Am. J. Physiol.* **213**: 1409–1413, 1967.

75. Hubel, K. A. The ins and outs of bicarbonate in the alimentary tract. *Gastroenterology* **54**: 647–651, 1968.

76. Islam, S., S. Reiser and P. A. Christiansen. Effect of thyroid hormones on the intestinal transport of valine in vitro. *Am. J. Dig. Dis.* **13**: 266–274, 1968.

77. Isselbacher, K. J., and J. R. Senior. The intestinal absorption of carbohydrate and fat. *Gastroenterology* **46**: 287–298, 1964.

78. Isselbacher, K. J. Biochemical aspects of fat absorption. *Gastroenterology* **50**: 78–82, 1966.

79. Isselbacher, K. J. Mechanisms of absorption of long and medium chain triglycerides. In: *Medium Chain Triglycerides.* Edited by J. R. Senior. Philadelphia: University of Pennsylvania Press, 1968, pp. 21–38.

80. Johnston, J. M. Mechanisms of fat absorption. In: *Handbook of Physiology.* Section 6: Alimentary Tract. Vol. III: Absorption. Edited by C. F. Code. Washington, D.C.: American Physiological Society, 1968, pp. 1353–1376.

81. Kayden, H. J., J. R. Senior, and F. H. Mattson. The monoglyceride pathway of fat absorption in man. *J. Clin. Invest.* **46**: 1695–1703, 1967.

82. Kaye, G. I., H. O. Wheeler, R. T. Whitlock, and N. Lane. Fluid transport in the rabbit gallbladder. *J. Cell. Biol.* **30**: 237–268, 1966.

83. Kershaw, T. G., K. D. Neame, and G. Wiseman. The effect of semi-starvation on absorption by the rat small intestine in vitro and in vivo. *J. Physiol.* **152**: 182–190, 1960.

84. Krawitt, E. L., and H. P. Schedl. In vivo calcium transport by rat small intestine. *Am. J. Physiol.* **214**: 232–236, 1968.

85. Lee, D. S., S. A. Hashim, and T. B. Van Itallie. Effect of long chain triglyceride on chylous transport of medium chain fatty acids. *Am. J. Physiol.* **214**: 294–297, 1968.

86. Lee, J. S., and K. M. Ducan. Lymphatic and venous transport of water from rat jejunum: a vascular perfusion study. *Gastroenterology* **54**: 559–567, 1968.

87. Lee, J. S. Isosmotic absorption of fluid from rat jejunum in vitro. *Gastroenterology* **54**: 366–374, 1968.

88. Levin, R. J. and D. H. Smyth. The effect of the thyroid gland on intestinal absorption of hexoses. *J. Physiol.* **169**: 755–769, 1963.

89. Levin, R. J. The effect of phloridzin on the potential difference and short circuit current of the large intestine. *Life Sci.* **5**: 1591–1596, 1966.

90. Levin, R. J., O. Koldovsky, J. Hoskova, V. Jirsova, and J. Uher. Electrical activity across human foetal small intestine associated with absorptive process. *Gut* **9**: 206–213, 1968.

91. Levin, R. J. Techniques, terminology and parameters in intestinal absorption. *Brit. Med. Bull.* **23**: 209–212, 1967.

92. Levitan, R., J. S. Fordtran, B. A. Burrows, and F. J. Inglefinger. Water and salt absorption in the human colon. *J. Clin. Invest.* **41**: 1754–1759, 1962.

93. Levitan, R., and F. J. Inglefinger. Effect of d-aldosterone on salt and water absorption from the intact human colon. *J. Clin. Invest.* **44:** 801–808, 1965.

94. Levitan, R., S. J. Malawer, and K. Goulston. Absorption of water and electrolytes from the human small bowel after d-aldosterone administration. *Fed. Proc.* **25:** 639, 1966.

95. Levitan, R., and K. Goulston. Water and electrolyte content of human ileostomy fluid after d-aldosterone administration. *Gastroenterology* **52:** 510–512, 1967.

96. Lifson, N., and A. A. Hakim. Simple diffusive-convective model for intestinal absorption of a non-electrolyte (urea). *Am. J. Physiol.* **211:** 1137–1146, 1966.

97. Lipkin, M. Cell proliferation in the gastrointestinal tract of man. *Fed. Proc.* **24:** 10–15, 1965.

98. Long, C. L., J. W. Geiger, and J. M. Kinney. Absorption of glucose from the colon and rectum. *Metabolism* **16:** 413–418, 1967.

99. Lowenstein, W. R., S. J. Socolar, S. Higashino, Y. Kanno, and N. Davidson. Intercellular communication: Renal, urinary bladder, sensory and salivary gland cells. *Science* **149:** 295–298, 1965.

100. McCleod, M. E., and M. P. Tyor. Transport of basic amino acids by hamster intestine. *Am. J. Physiol.* **213:** 163–168, 1967.

101. McConnell, K. P., and G. J. Cho. Active transport of L-selenomethionine in the intestine. *Am. J. Physiol.* **213:** 150–156, 1967.

102. McMichael, H. B., J. Webb, and A. M. Dawson. The absorption of maltose and lactose in man. *Clin. Sci.* **33:** 135–145, 1967.

103. Matthews, D. M., and L. Laster. Absorption of protein digestion products: A review. *Gut* **6:** 411–426, 1965.

104. Matthews, D. M. Absorption of water-soluble vitamins. *Brit. Med. Bull.* **23:** 258–262, 1967.

105. Morris, I. G. Gammaglobulin absorption in newborn. In: *Handbook of Physiology.* Section 6: Alimentary Tract. Vol. III: Absorption. Edited by C. F. Code. Washington, D.C.: American Physiological Society, 1968, pp. 1491–1512.

106. Mossberg, S. M. Ammonia absorption in hamster ileum: Effect of pH and total CO_2 on transport in everted sacs. *Am. J. Physiol.* **213:** 1327–1330, 1967.

107. Munro, H. N. Protein secretion into the gastrointestinal tract. In: *Postgraduate Gastroenterology.* Edited by T. J. Thomson and I. E. Gillespie. London: Bailliere, Tindall and Cassell, 1966, pp. 58–67.

108. Newey, H., P. A. Sanford, and D. H. Smyth. Some effects of ouabain and potassium on transport and metabolism in rat small intestine. *J. Physiol.* **194:** 237–248, 1968.

109. Nordin, B. E. C. Measurement and meaning of calcium absorption. *Gastroenterology* **54:** 294–301, 1968.

110. Nunn, A. S., Jr., and M. S. Ellert. Absorption and electrolyte changes of intestinal mucosa following substrate induction. *Am. J. Physiol.* **212:** 711–716, 1967.

111. Olsen, W. A., and F. J. Inglefinger. The role of sodium in intestinal glucose absorption in man. *J. Clin. Invest.* **47:** 1133–1142, 1968.

112. Onstad, G. R., L. J. Schoenfield, and J. A. Higgins. Fluid transfer in the everted human gallbladder. *J. Clin. Invest.* **46:** 606–614, 1967.

113. Ostrow, J. D. Absorption of bile pigments by the gall bladder. *J. Clin. Invest.* **46:** 2035–2052, 1967.

114. Parsons, D. S. Salt and water absorption by the intestinal tract. *Brit. Med. Bull.* **23:** 252–257, 1967.

115. Parsons, D. S. Methods for investigation of intestinal absorption. In: *The Handbook of Physiology*. Section 6: Alimentary Tract. Vol. III: Absorption. Edited by C. F. Code. Washington, D.C.: American Physiological Society, 1968, pp. 1177–1216.

116. Pearse, A. G. E., and E. O. Riecken. Histology and cytochemistry of cells of small intestine in relation to absorption. *Brit. Med. Bull.* 23: 217–222, 1967.

117. Peters, C. J., and M. Walser. Transport of cations by rabbit gallbladder: Evidence suggesting a common cation pump. *Am. J. Physiol.* 210: 677–683, 1966.

118. Phillips, S. F., and C. F. Code. Sorption of potassium in the small and large intestine. *Am. J. Physiol.* 211: 607–613, 1966.

119. Phillips, S. F., and W. H. J. Summerskill. Comparison of electrolyte transport in relation to intraluminal concentrations in the human jejunum and ileum. *J. Clin. Invest.* 45: 1056, 1966.

120. Playoust, M. R., and K. J. Isselbacher. Studies on the intestinal absorption and intramucosal lipolysis of a medium chain triglyceride. *J. Clin. Invest.* 43: 878–885, 1964.

121. Rampone, A. J. Cholesterol absorption using chromic oxide in an indicator ratio method. *Am. J. Physiol.* 214: 1370–1373, 1968.

122. Reeve, J., and J. J. Franks. Fatty acid synthesis by jejunal slices from rats fed medium and long chain triglycerides. *Am. J. Physiol.* 214: 1425–1428, 1968.

123. Reynell, P. C., and G. H. Spray. The absorption of glucose by the intact rat. *J. Physiol.* 134: 531–537, 1956.

124. Reiser, S., and P. A. Christiansen. Intestinal transport of valine as affected by ionic environment. *Am. J. Physiol.* 212: 1297–1302, 1967.

125. Rodgers, J. B., E. M. Riley, G. D. Drummey, and K. J. Isselbacher. Lipid absorption in adrenalectomized rats: The role of altered enzyme activity in the intestinal mucosa. *Gastroenterology* 53: 547–556, 1967.

126. Rosenberg, L. E., J. C. Crawhall, and S. Segal. Intestinal transport of cystine and cysteine in man: Evidence for separate mechanisms. *J. Clin. Invest.* 46: 30–34, 1967.

127. Saunders, S. J., and K. J. Isselbacher. Intestinal absorption of amino acids. *Gastroenterology* 50: 586–595, 1966.

128. Schachter, D., E. B. Dowdle, and H. Schenker. Active transport of calcium by the small intestine of the rat. *Am. J. Physiol.* 198: 263–268, 1960.

129. Schachter, D., S. Kowarski, J. D. Finkelstein, and R. W. Ma. Tissue concentration differences during active transport of calcium by intestine. *Am. J. Physiol.* 211: 1131–1136, 1966.

130. Scholer, J. F., and C. F. Code. Rate of absorption of water from stomach and small bowel of human beings. *Gastroenterology* 27: 565–577, 1954.

131. Schedl, H. P., and J. A. Clifton. Cortisol absorption in man. *Gastroenterology* 44: 134–145, 1963.

132. Schedl, H. P., C. E. Pierce, A. Rider, and J. A. Clifton. Absorption of L-methionine from the human small intestine. *J. Clin. Invest.* 47: 417–425, 1968.

133. Schedl, H. P., G. W. Osbaldison, and I. H. Mills. Absorption secretion and precipitation of calcium in the small intestine of the dog. *Am. J. Physiol.* 214: 814–819, 1968.

134. Schulz, S. G., and P. F. Curran. Intestinal absorption of sodium chloride. In: *Handbook of Physiology*. Section 6: Alimentary Tract. Vol. III: Absorption.

Edited by C. F. Code. Washington, D.C.: American Physiological Society, 1968, pp. 1245–1276.

135. Schwabe, A. D., V. D. Valdivieso, S. Merrill, C. Ortega, L. R. Bennett, and J. C. Thompson. Studies on the intestinal absorption of a medium chain fat (trioctanoin) in normal and pancreatectomized dogs. *Am. J. Digest. Dis.* **12:** 1114–1121, 1967.

136. Semenza, G., R. Tosi, M. C. Vallotton-Delachaux, and E. Mulhaupt. Sodium activation of human intestinal sucrase and its possible significance in the enzymatic organization of brush borders. *Biochim. Biophys. Acta.* **89:** 109–116, 1964.

137. Senior, J. R., and K. J. Isselbacher. Demonstration of an intestinal monoglyceride lipase: An enzyme with a possible role in intracellular completion of fat digestion. *J. Clin. Invest.* **42:** 187–195, 1963.

138. Senior, J. R. Intestinal absorption of fats. *J. Lipid Res.* **5:** 495–521, 1964.

139. Shah, B. G., and H. H. Draper. Depression of calcium absorption in parathyroidectomized rats. *Am. J. Physiol.* **211:** 963–966, 1966.

140. Smyth, D. H. Intestinal absorption. In: *Recent Advances in Physiology* (8th ed.). Edited by R. Creese. Boston: Little, Brown & Co., 1963, pp. 36–68.

141. Strauss, E. W. Morphological aspects of triglyceride absorption. In: *Handbook of Physiology.* Section 6: Alimentary Tract. Vol. III: Absorption. Edited by C. F. Code. Washington D.C.: American Physiological Society, 1968, pp. 1377–1406.

142. Swallow, J. H., and C. F. Code. Intestinal transmucosal fluxes of bicarbonate. *Am. J. Physiol.* **212:** 717–723, 1967.

143. Taylor, A. E., E. M. Wright, S. G. Schultz, and P. F. Curran. Effect of sugars on ion fluxes in intestine. *Am. J. Physiol.* **214:** 836–842, 1968.

144. Tidball, C. S., and M. E. Tidball. Changes in net absorption of a NaCl solution produced by atropine in normal and vagotomized dogs. *Am. J. Physiol.* **193:** 25–28, 1958.

145. Treadwell, C. R., and G. V. Vahouny. Cholesterol absorption. In: *Handbook of Physiology.* Section 6: Alimentary Tract. Vol. III: Absorption. Edited by C. F. Code. Washington, D.C.: American Physiological Society, 1968, pp. 1407–1438.

146. Trier, J. S. Morphology of the epithelium of the small intestine. In: *Handbook of Physiology.* Section 6: Alimentary Tract. Vol III: Absorption. Edited by C. F. Code. Washington, D.C.: American Physiological Society, 1968, pp. 1125–1176.

147. Vinnik, I. E., F. Kern, Jr., and K. E. Sussman. The effect of diabetes mellitus and insulin on glucose absorption by the small intestine in man. *J. Lab. Clin. Med.* **66:** 131–136, 1965.

148. Visscher, M. B. Transport of water and electrolyte across intestinal epithelia. In: *Metabolic Aspects of Transport Across Cell Membranes.* Edited by Q. R. Murphy. Madison: University of Wisconsin Press, 1957, pp. 57–71.

149. Weiner, I. M., and L. Lack. Bile salt absorption: Enterohepatic circulation. In: *Handbook of Physiology.* Section 6: Alimentary Tract. Vol. III: Absorption. Edited by C. F. Code. Washington, D.C.: American Physiological Society, 1968, pp. 1439–1456.

150. Wheeler, H. O. Transport of electrolytes and water across wall of rabbit gall bladder. *Am. J. Physiol.* **205:** 427–438, 1963.

151. Whitlock, R. T., and H. O. Wheeler. Coupled transport of solute and water across rabbit gallbladder epithelium. *J. Clin. Invest.* **43:** 2249–2265, 1964.

152. Whitlock, R. T., and H. O. Wheeler. Anion transport by isolated rabbit gallbladders. *Am. J. Physiol.* **213:** 1199–1204, 1967.
153. Williams, A. W. Electron microscopic changes associated with water absorption in the jejunum. *Gut* **4:** 1–7, 1963.
154. Wilson, J. D. Biosynthetic origin of serum cholesterol in the squirrel monkey: Evidence for a contribution by the intestinal wall. *J. Clin. Invest.* **47:** 175–187, 1968.
155. Wilson, T. H. *Intestinal Absorption.* Philadelphia: W. B. Saunders Co., 1962.
156. Wilson, T. H. Intestinal absorption of vitamin B_{12}. *Physiologist* **6:** 11–26, 1963.
157. Wilson, T. H. Structure and function of the intestinal absorptive cell. In: *The Cellular Function of Membrane Transport.* Edited by J. F. Hoffman. Englewood Cliffs, N.J.: Prentice-Hall, 1964, pp. 215–229.
158. Wiseman, G. Absorption of amino acids. In: *Handbook of Physiology.* Section 6: Alimentary Tract. Vol. III: Absorption. Edited by C. F. Code. Washington, D.C.: American Physiological Society, 1968, pp. 1277–1309.
159. Wiseman, G. *Absorption from the Intestine.* New York: Academic Press, 1964.
160. Zilversmit, D. B. The composition and structure of lymph chylomicrons in dog, rat and man. *J. Clin. Invest.* **44:** 1610–1622, 1965.

Additional Reading

Absorption, Vol. III. *Handbook of Physiology.* Section 6: Alimentary Tract. Washington, D.C.: American Physiological Society, 1968.
Intestinal absorption. *Brit. Med. Bull.* 23: 1967.
Wilson, T. H. *Intestinal Absorption.* Philadelphia: W. B. Saunders Co., 1962.
Wiseman, G. *Absorption from the Intestine.* New York: Academic Press, 1964.

CHAPTER

Motor Function of the Gastrointestinal Tract

THE PHYSIOLOGY OF THE GUT as a conduit for the intestinal stream is the least satisfactorily understood function of the gastrointestinal tract. There is indeed no generally acceptable term for this function. *Motility* is used widely but is difficult to define. *Motor function* may be a temporarily satisfactory term. Motor function may be studied from a variety of viewpoints—the physiology of smooth muscle, the peristaltic reflex of an isolated segment of intestine, pressures within isolated intestinal loops in anesthetized animals, or the behavior of specific portions of the gastrointestinal tract of conscious man recorded by pressure-sensing telemetering devices. The physiology of smooth muscle has strong relationships to pharmacology and biochemistry and has shared with these disciplines in the popularity of "molecular biology." The investigator of motor function in intact organisms has tended to become a prisoner of his technique—balloons, open-tipped catheters, or cineradiography. The precise relationships between the results recorded by these devices and the properties of the gut responsible for its normal function are only now being investigated by simultaneous recordings with multiple techniques (22).

Structural Features of Smooth Muscle

It is clear that the absence of cross striations in muscle fibers is characteristic of muscle in a variety of organs with rather sharply different physiologic properties. Therefore it is prudent to specify smooth muscle of the intestine. Furthermore, there are significant species differences, and differences between smooth muscle in various parts of the gastrointestinal tract. Much of the recent work on the physiology of smooth muscle has been done on the taenia coli of the guinea pig because it can be obtained free of nerve cells and handled easily in vitro. However, guinea pig intestine has a number of exceptional characteristics, and generalizations to human intestinal muscle in vivo may not be warranted.

Smooth muscle cells are spindle-shaped cells with discrete borders rather than a syncitium. The true length of the cells in vivo is unknown, but it is probably less than 250 μ (19). The filaments are of one size only and have the same diameter as actin filaments of striated muscle. Using permanganate fixation, Dewey and Barr (18,19) found areas of fusion between the outer membranes of adjacent cell membranes. They gave the term *nexus* to these structures. Fusion of the outer dense layer of the cell membranes probably involves noncarbohydrate moieties. The carbohydrate-containing layer does not participate. When the tissue is soaked in hypertonic solutions, the nexuses rupture.

In some species the cell membranes form bulbous projections into adjacent cells. The fact that the myofibrils were oriented obliquely to the long axis of muscle fibers and inserted along the side of fibers increases the number of elements in parallel rather than in series. This permitted a fourfold increase in tension in the longitudinal direction (37).

The major significance of the nexus is that it may provide the explanation for the mechanism of conduction between muscle cells. Such a low-resistance pathway would explain the spread of electrical excitation through muscle in the fashion of a syncitium. Spread by mechanical deformation seemed unlikely, since conduction occurred with the muscle immobilized (33). It was not blocked or potentiated by drugs. As a result of these considerations, conduction was judged to be of an electrical rather than a chemical nature. Barr provided direct evidence for conduction between cells using the sucrose-gap technique of recording with microelectrodes (2). Spread of activity down the intact intestine is from side-to-side and due to bundle-to-bundle conduction rather than cell-to-cell. Excitation proceeds faster in some bundles than in others (3). Transmission is best when the muscle has been made excitable by stretch or chemical transmitters (12). The space between fibers within bundles has been estimated at 9 to 12.5 per cent (32). Intercellular distances vary widely in different smooth muscles.

Properties of Intestinal Smooth Muscle

Perhaps the most striking feature of the muscle of the wall of the intestine is its ability to vary its length with minimal changes in tension. Length may increase several times the minimal length (26). Contraction times are long but relaxation times are even longer. Oxygen consumption does increase with increase in tension but values remain low (9). The oxygen consumption of spontaneously active taenia coli was only one-fourth that of striated muscle at rest. The second feature of intestinal smooth muscle is its property of spontaneous rhythmic activity. The behavior of the rabbit intestine in vitro is a frequent laboratory exercise. The ability of this tissue to exhibit a monotonous sine wave of phasic activity is dear to the heart of laboratory instructors. More elegant preparations such as the taenia coli or embryonic intestinal smooth muscle before the development of innervation, show that the property of rhythmic contraction resides in the muscle cells alone.

In recent years it is the electrical properties of smooth muscle that have received the most attention (15). Three types of changes in membrane potentials have been recognized—prepotentials, slow waves, and spikes. The resting membrane potential varies in amplitude, depending upon the technique of recording. In general it has been around 50 mv in taenia coli (10). Since the cells are spontaneously active it is difficult to obtain a steady value. With excitation, the cell depolarizes. This may or may not result in a reversal of polarity. Figure 10-1 illustrates spikes in which the cell was acting as a pacemaker and exhibits a prepotential. For comparison a neighboring cell was excited by spread from the first and shows no prepotential. It is a "driven" cell (26). The variability of recordings of spikes involves elements of both membrane potential and membrane current (6).

With extracellular recordings from intestinal wall, a characteristic positive wave lasting two to three seconds can be recorded. On the descending limb, spike activity may occur and, coincident with it, mechanical contraction of

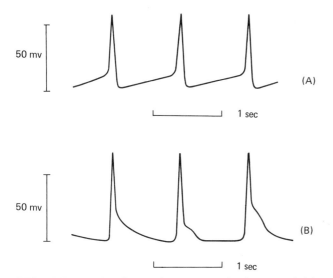

FIGURE 10-1.   Contrasting patterns of activity recorded from the taenia coli (guinea pig). A: Characteristic of a "pacemaker"; B: Characteristic of a "driven" cell. (From M. E. Holman. In: *Handbook of Physiology*. Section 6: Alimentary Tract. Vol. IV. Edited by C. F. Code. Washington, D.C.: American Physiological Society, 1968, p. 1687.)

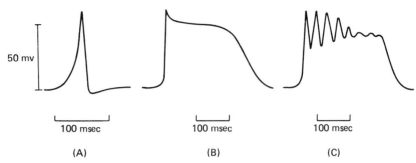

50 mv

100 msec   100 msec   100 msec

(A)   (B)   (C)

FIGURE 10-2.   Three different forms of action potential recorded from visceral smooth muscles. (From M. E. Holman. In: *Handbook of Physiology*. Section 6: Alimentary Tract. Vol. IV. Edited by C. F. Code. Washington, D.C.: American Physiological Society, 1968, p. 1681.)

the intestine. Figure 10-2 is an example. Studies of individual muscle layers showed that the slow wave was derived from the longitudinal muscle and spread secondarily to circular muscle (27). The slow waves can be influenced by local reflexes, temperature, and hypoxia but not by anticholinergic drugs. Slow waves spread synchronously around the gut. They have been regarded as a manifestation of a trigger mechanism for contraction.

The slow waves in the stomach are somewhat more complex, consisting of an initial positive deflection which is propagated and a slower second potential which is not propagated but can be correlated with contraction (17,31). Figure 10-3 illustrates this type of electrical activity. Spikes may occur on the second component. The initial potential is analagous to intestinal slow waves and the second to prepotentials (31).

The frequency of slow waves is characteristic for the area of the intestinal tract. In the stomach they occur at the rate of 4 to 5/min in dogs (16). In the duodenum the rate is 18/min, decreasing to about 11 in the ileum. Cutting or clamping the intestine results in an abrupt slowing of the rate of slow waves distal to the section. The term *basic electrical rhythm* has been given to the slow waves (4). They may play an important role in the gradient of activity in the intestine which decreases from duodenum to ileum and contributes to the aboral passage of intestinal content. Waxing and waning of slow-wave activity can be seen in segments of intestine (34). This may represent zones of overlap between pacemakers (20). Daniel and Irwin suggested that, in the stomach, the duodenal electrical activity may represent a 3:1 or 4:1 harmonic of gastric activity (17). Slow waves are reduced in the absence of sodium or by ouabain. Prepotentials are more sensitive to calcium (34).

Electrolyte Composition of Smooth Muscle

In general intestinal smooth muscle contains potassium in lower and sodium in higher concentrations than striated muscle (11). The extracellular

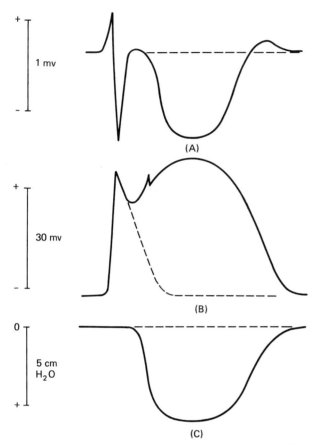

FIGURE 10-3. Diagrammatic representation of electrical and mechanical recordings from the antrum of the active stomach. A: Extracellular recording; B: Intracellular recording. C: Pressure in luminal balloon. Calibrations as shown. Each antral complex lasts about 12 seconds. Dashed line shows for comparison the recordings from the inactive stomach. (From E. E. Daniel and J. Irwin. Electrical activity of gastric musculature. In: *Handbook of Physiology.* Section 6: Alimentary Tract. Vol. IV: Motility. Edited by C. F. Code. Washington, D.C.: American Physiological Society, 1968, pp. 1969–1984.)

space is relatively large in smooth muscle (*24*). The intracellular space is not homogeneous. At least two compartments exist for D_2O, of which the slowest equilibration occurs with the nucleus and mitochondria (*42*). Calcium also exists in bound and free form, the latter in concentration related linearly to that in the external medium (*11*).

Ionic Basis of Action Potentials

Coincident with the action potential there is a rapid entrance of sodium and a slow exit of potassium (*11,28*). Calcium probably activates the contractile mechanism during the action potential and is derived from a calcium pool associated with cell membranes (26). The height of the spike depends upon the calcium concentration in the medium (11). Calcium uptake increases during contraction (24,1). Barium chloride increased the frequency of spontaneous spike discharge with no effect on resting potential (39).

When the taenia coli of the guinea pig is placed under stretch, the membrane potential falls and the frequency of the variations in potentials increases. Bulbring suggested that deformation of smooth muscle cells may lead to changes in membrane permeability and hence the change in potential (11). She also showed that the membrane potential was directly related to tension but not to the length of the muscle.

Contractile Proteins of Smooth Muscle

The myosin of intestinal smooth muscle differs in its amino acid composition from that in striated muscle (30). No myosin filaments can be seen, and the endoplasmic reticulum is poorly developed (14). Small myosin aggregates can be extracted as dimers in dispersed form. Contraction may be associated with combination of actin with these aggregates. Glycogenolysis is also a concomitant of contraction (29).

Control of Smooth Muscle

The functional unit of intestinal smooth muscle is a group of smooth muscle cells. Single cells in the taenia coli do not initiate an action potential in response to stimulation via an intracellular electrode. The functional unit probably includes 12 cells in a hexagonal bundle (5). Nerve bundles approach within 200 to 1,000 Å from the nearest smooth muscle cell. In rats, vesiculated nerve processes orient themselves to the long axis of smooth muscle cells and may fit into a depression on the surface of the cells (40). Vesicles were seen on opposite sides in both nerve ending and smooth muscle cell. The plasma membranes were about 80 Å in thickness and contained both vesicles and mitochondria. In amphibians, multiple axons can be seen in contact with smooth muscle cells (36,41).

The ability to identify norepinephrine by fluorescent stains permitted the description of varicosities along the course of sympathetic adrenergic neurons containing the transmitter (25). Inhibition of smooth muscle contraction can occur by stimulation of perivascular sympathetic fibers or by intramural nerves with their ganglion cells in the myenteric plexus (13). The transmitter in the latter case is unknown. The distribution of norepinephrine about ganglion cells in the myenteric plexus suggests that inhibition may be exerted at the ganglion level rather than upon smooth muscle cells directly.

Bulbring considered that the submucosal plexus was largely concerned with sensory function, while the myenteric plexus was predominantly motor (9). Action potentials are not necessary for contraction in response to acetylcholine or for inhibition with norepinephrine, although both probably occur under normal circumstances (38). There is much speculation that relaxation in response to norepinephrine may involve cylic AMP (8,21). Paton's theory that it is the rate of turnover at receptor sites rather than occupation per se that determines drug action may be helpful in explaining the action of chemical transmission (35).

Smooth Muscle of the Intestine in Man

Human taenia coli responded to acetylcholine by contraction, while norepinephrine and isoprenaline inhibited spontaneous activity (7). Beta blockers prevented the inhibitory action. There was no evidence of parasympathetic innervation of the colon in man (23). Nicotine produced relaxation, while physostigmine was without effect. These results would support the role of sympathetic inhibition in the control of human colonic muscle and minimize the role of the parasympathetics.

Pathophysiology

As yet the large amount of information on the physiology of smooth muscle has had little application to human disease. Slow waves can be used as a means of studying the spread of excitation. Parasympathomimetic drugs are used to stimulate activity of the intestine after surgery, and anticholinergics are used as antispasmodics to relax contractile segments of the intestine.

References

1. Banerjee, A. K., and J. J. Lewis. Influence of drugs upon $^{47}Ca^{2+}$ uptake in depolarized intestinal smooth muscle. *J. Pharm. Pharmacol.* **16:** 439–440, 1964.
2. Barr, L. Transmembrane resistance of smooth muscle cells. *Am. J. Physiol.* **200:** 1251–1255, 1961.
3. Barr, L., and M. M. Dewey. Electrotonus and electrical transmission in smooth muscle. In: *Handbook of Physiology.* Section 6: Alimentary Tract. Vol. IV: Motility. Edited by C. F. Code. Washington, D.C.: American Physiological Society, 1968, pp. 1733–1742.
4. Bass, P. Electrical activity of smooth muscle of the gastrointestinal tract. *Gastroenterology* **49:** 391–394, 1965.

5. Bennett, M. R., and G. Burnstock. Electrophysiology of the innervation of intestinal smooth muscle. In: *Handbook of Physiology*. Section 6: Alimentary Tract. Vol. IV: Motility. Edited by C. F. Code. Washington, D.C.: American Physiological Society, 1968, pp. 1709–1732.

6. Bortoff, A. Configuration of intestinal slow waves obtained by monopolar recording techniques. *Am. J. Physiol.* **213:** 157–162, 1967.

7. Bucknell, A. and B. Whitney. A preliminary investigation of the pharmacology of the human isolated taenia coli preparation. *Brit. J. Pharmacol.* **23:** 164–175, 1964.

8. Bueding, E., R. W. Butcher, J. Hawkins, A. R. Timms, and E. W. Sutherland, Jr. Effect of epinephrine on cyclic adenosine 3'5' phosphate and hexose phosphates in intestinal smooth muscle. *Biochim. Biophys. Acta.* **115:** 173–178, 1966.

9. Bulbring, E. The action of humoral transmitters on smooth muscle. *Brit. Med. Bull.* **13:** 172–175, 1957.

10. Bulbring, E. Smooth muscle of the alimentary tract. In: *Modern Trends in Gastroenterology*. Second Series. Edited by F. Avery Jones. New York: Paul B. Hoeber Inc., 1958, pp. 1–11.

11. Bulbring, E. Electrical activity in intestinal smooth muscle. *Physiol. Rev. Suppl.* **42:** 160–178, 1962.

12. Burnstock, G., and C. L. Prosser. Conduction in smooth muscles: Comparative electrical properties. *Am. J. Physiol.* **199:** 553–559, 1960.

13. Burnstock, G., G. Campbell, and M. J. Rand. The inhibitory innervation of the taenia of the guinea pig caecum. *J. Physiol. (London)* **182:** 504–526, 1966.

14. Casteels, R. The physiology of intestinal smooth muscle. *Am. J. Dig. Dis.* **12:** 231–236, 1967.

15. Daniel, E. E., A. J. Honour, and A. Bogoch. Electrical activity of the longitudinal muscle of dog small intestine studied in vivo using microelectrodes. *Am. J. Physiol.* **198:** 113–118, 1960.

16. Daniel, E. E. The electrical and contractile activity of the pyloric region in dogs and the effects of drugs. *Gastroenterology* **49:** 403–418, 1965.

17. Daniel, E. E., and J. Irwin. Electrical activity of gastric musculature. In: *Handbook of Physiology*. Section 6: Alimentary Tract. Vol. IV: Motility. Edited by C. F. Code. Washington, D.C.: American Physiological Society, 1968, pp. 1969–1984.

18. Dewey, M. M. The anatomical basis of propagation in smooth muscle. *Gastroenterology* **49:** 395–402, 1965.

19. Dewey, M. M., and L. Barr. Structure of vertebrate intestinal smooth muscle. In: *Handbook of Physiology*. Section 6: Alimentary Tract. Vol. IV: Motility. Edited by C. F. Code. Washington, D.C.: American Physiological Society, 1968, pp. 1629–1654.

20. Diamant, N. E., and A. Bortoff. Intestinal slow wave frequency gradient. *Fed. Proc.* **27:** 449, 1968.

21. Diamond, J., and T. M. Brody. Effect of catecholamines on smooth muscle motility and phosphorylase activity. *J. Pharmacol. Exp. Ther.* **152:** 202–220, 1966.

22. Farrar, J. T. Gastrointestinal smooth muscle function. *Am. J. Dig. Dis.* **8:** 103–110, 1963.

23. Fishlock, D. J., and A. G. Parks. The action of nicotine on the circular muscle of the human ileum and colon in vitro. *Brit. J. Pharmacol.* **26:** 79–86, 1966.

24. Goodford, P. J. Distribution and exchange of electrolytes in intestinal smooth muscle. In: *Handbook of Physiology.* Section 6: Alimentary Tract. Vol. IV: Motility. Edited by C. F. Code. Washington, D.C.: American Physiological Society, 1968, pp. 1743–1766.

25. Hillarp, N. A. The construction and functional organization of the autonomic innervation apparatus. *Acta Physiol. Scand.* **46:** Suppl. 157, 1959, pp. 1–38.

26. Holman, M. E. Introduction to electrophysiology of visceral smooth muscle. In: *Handbook of Physiology.* Section 6: Alimentary Tract. Vol. IV: Motility. Edited by C. F. Code. Washington, D.C.: American Physiological Society, 1968, pp. 1665–1708.

27. Kobayashi, M., T. Nagai, and C. L. Prosser. Electrical interaction between muscle layers of cat intestine. *Am. J. Physiol.* **211:** 1281–1291, 1966.

28. Kuriyama, H. Ionic basis of smooth muscle action potentials. In: *Handbook of Physiology.* Section 6: Alimentary Tract. Vol. IV: Motility. Edited by C. F. Code. Washington, D.C.: American Physiological Society, 1968, pp. 1767–1791.

29. Lundholm, L., and E. Mohme-Lundholm. Contraction and glycogenolysis of smooth muscle. *Acta Physiol. Scand.* **57:** 125–129, 1963.

30. Needham, D. M., and C. F. Shoenberg. Proteins of the contractile mechanism in vertebrate smooth muscle. In: *Handbook of Physiology.* Section 6: Alimentary Tract. Vol. IV: Motility. Edited by C. F. Code. Washington, D.C.: American Physiological Society, 1968, pp. 1793–1810.

31. Papasova, M. P., T. Nagai, and C. L. Prosser. Two-component slow waves in smooth muscle of cat stomach. *Am. J. Physiol.* **214:** 695–702, 1968.

32. Prosser, C. L., G. Burnstock, and J. Kahn. Conduction in smooth muscle: Comparative structural properties. *Am. J. Physiol.* **199:** 545–552, 1960.

33. Prosser, C. L. Introduction to symposium on gastrointestinal smooth muscle. *Gastroenterology* **49:** 389–390, 1965.

34. Prosser, C. L., and A. Bortoff. Electrical activity of intestinal muscle under in vitro conditions. In: *Handbook of Physiology.* Section 6: Alimentary Tract. Vol. IV: Motility. Edited by C. F. Code. Washington, D.C.: American Physiological Society, 1968, pp. 2025–2050.

35. Rang, H. P. The pharmacology of intestinal smooth muscle. *Am. J. Digest. Dis.* **12:** 237–244, 1967.

36. Rogers, D. C., and G. Burnstock. Multiaxonal autonomic junctions in intestinal smooth muscle of the toad (*Bufus marinus*). *J. Comp. Neurol.* **126:** 625–651, 1966.

37. Rosenbluth, J. Smooth muscle: An ultrastructural basis for the dynamics of its contraction. *Science* **148:** 1337–1339, 1965.

38. Schatzmann, H. J. Action of acetylcholine and epinephrine on intestinal smooth muscle. In: *Handbook of Physiology.* Section 6: Alimentary Tract. Vol. IV: Motility. Edited by C. F. Code. Washington, D.C.: American Physiological Society: 1968, pp. 2173–2191.

39. Suzuki, T., A. Nishiyama, and K. Okamura. The effects of barium ion on the resting and action potential of intestinal smooth muscle cell. *Tohoku J. Exp. Med.* **82:** 87–92, 1964.

40. Thaemert, J. C. The ultrastructure and disposition of vesiculated nerve processes in smooth muscle. *J. Cell Biol.* **16:** 361–377, 1963.

41. Thaemert, J. C. Ultrastructural interrelationships of nerve processes and smooth muscle cells in three dimensions. *J. Cell Biol.* **28:** 37–49, 1966.

42. Weiner, D. E., and E. Grim. Kinetics of distribution of D_2O in canine intestinal tissues. *Am. J. Physiol.* **211:** 600–606, 1966.

Additional Reading

Motility, Vol. IV. *Handbook of Physiology,* Section 6: Alimentary Tract. Washington, D.C.: American Physiological Society, 1968.

Esophageal Motility

THE ESOPHAGUS is a conduit for the conduction of liquids and solids from the mouth and pharynx to the stomach. This is accomplished in part by the force of gravity and by progressive waves of contraction sweeping down from the aortic arch to the diaphragm, the prime example of peristalsis in the gastrointestinal tract. Normal function demands that the airway be protected from food and the lower end of the esophagus from regurgitation of acid-pepsin. This is accomplished in part by sphincter mechanisms at the upper and lower ends of the esophagus. During swallowing the sphincters relax in a coordinated fashion to permit passage of the bolus. The extrinsic nerves participate in this act.

Since it is accessible with minimal difficulty, the esophagus has been a favored area of study of motility. Balloons, catheters connected to strain gauges outside the patient, miniature transducers, and cineradiography have been applied to the study of the esophagus. The human subject lends himself to this kind of investigation. Furthermore, the cat is the only commonly used laboratory animal with a comparable muscular structure of the esophagus.

Structure of the Esophagus

The human esophagus consists of a hollow tube with a distinct muscular constriction at the upper end, the cricopharyngeus, and a lower end with debatable evidence of a muscular sphincter (29). The proximal third of the wall consists of striated muscle, the middle third of mixed striated and smooth muscle, and the lower third of smooth muscle. In most laboratory animals the entire esophagus is supplied by striated muscle (11). The mucosa is covered by stratified squamous epithelium. A matter of considerable importance is the definition of the junction between the esophagus and the stomach. Unfortunately there is no easy solution. The junction between stratified squamous epithelium of the esophagus and columnar epithelium of the stomach is an irregular zone which is not constantly related to the diaphragmatic hiatus or various structures seen by the radiologist at the lower end of the esophagus. The confusion of terms has made it difficult for specialists in the various disciplines to communicate with each other.

The radiologic anatomy of the lower end of the esophagus is based upon the diaphragmatic hiatus and the appearance of mucosal folds in the stomach and esophagus. In addition, many subjects show a narrow band of constriction of minor degree above the diaphragm, commonly described as a ring (51). Proximal to this, a dilatation of the esophagus of variable degree may be seen. It is particularly prominent after swallowing barium and taking a deep inspiration. This is the phrenic ampulla. During deep inspiration, passage of barium into the stomach is often interrupted, and the ampulla can be seen to empty in a retrograde fashion into the body of the esophagus (50). Figure 11-1 is an illustration of the anatomy of the lower end of the esophagus. Suffice it to say, it may be difficult for the radiologist to define the esophagogastric junction and to make the diagnosis of hiatal hernia—protrusion of a portion of the stomach through the diaphragmatic hiatus.

Various structures have been thought to contribute to the competence of the sphincter mechanism at the lower end of the esophagus. The diaphragm itself, the angle of relation between the fundus of the stomach and the esophagus, and the phrenicoesophageal ligament have been implicated (32). Many of the experiments have been done on dogs, and their significance for man is uncertain. According to Atkinson, resistance to reflux from the stomach into the esophagus is low (5 cm H_2O) in the cadaver and coincidentally the usual angle between the esophagus and stomach is lost (3). Increased intraabdominal pressure applied by external compression did not alter the pressure gradient across the esophagogastric junction, but deep inspiration did have an effect compatible with a pinchcock mechanism (46).

Physiologic evidence for the esophagogastric junction includes a high-pressure zone and a change in the transmucosal potential difference (PD). In the stomach the mucosa is negative with respect to an indifferent electrode, while the difference is lost in the esophagus. When the high-pressure zone was correlated with the change in PD, a good agreement was obtained (31). The change in PD was related to the appearance of biopsies of mucosa. Above the area of change, no parietal cells could be identified. In most subjects, stratified squamous epithelium was present, but in some, columnar epithelium could be recognized.

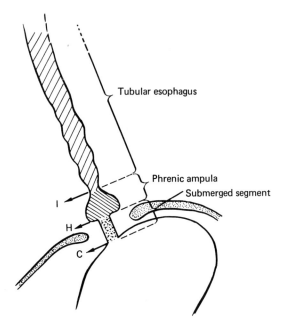

FIGURE 11-1. The main divisions of the "gullet" or tube which extends from the cricopharynx to the stomach. This tube may be divided, at least for roentgen purposes, into three main parts, two above the hiatus consist of the tubular esophagus which extends from this point to the hiatus. The third division is the "submerged segment." The inferior esophageal sphincter (I), an intrinsic landmark, marks the junction between the tubular esophagus and the phrenic ampula. The hiatus of the diaphragm (H), an extrinsic landmark, indicates the junction between the phrenic ampula of the submerged segment. The cardia or cardiac orifice (C) is at the junction of the submerged segment with the saclike stomach. This illustration is purely diagrammatic since there is no normal functional phase that shows continuous filling of the three divisions in this fashion. (From B. S. Wolf: *Amer. J. Dig. Dis.* **5:** 751–769, 1960.)

Characteristics of Esophageal Motility

The motor activity of the body of the esophagus is usually recorded by passing open-tipped catheters into the esophagus and connecting them to strain gauges outside the body. The catheters may or may not be flushed by a slow continuous flow of saline. Commonly three catheters are bound together with their tips 5 cm apart (*11*). Code and his associates have made use of miniature transducers intoduced into the esophagus, but they require a considerable degree of sophistication for operation and maintenance (*6*).

As an independent technique or for simultaneous studies, cineradiography can be used to record the movements of the barium-filled esophagus on motion-picture film (*12*). With either procedure, investigators agree that the most prominent feature of esophageal motor activity is a contraction of large amplitude which passes from the upper esophagus to the lower end in response to swallowing (10,11,27). Figure 11-2 is an example of the manometric characteristics of this contraction, known as the primary peristaltic wave. Attempts at refinement of recordings have brought controversy. Butin et al. reported an initial negative pressure deflection followed by three positive waves, the last of which was the peristaltic wave (6). However, one or more of these waves was absent in two thirds of their subjects. Other investigators have failed to detect initial negative waves, and the first positive wave may be absent with "dry swallows." In a variable percentage of subjects, primary peristaltic waves do not follow swallowing. Kantrowitz et al. found that peristaltic waves occurred after 76 to 100 per cent of swallows (28). In the aged, this fell to 50 per cent (43).

A similar manometric event can be produced by inflating a balloon in the midesophagus without swallowing—so-called secondary peristalsis (15,40). The incidence of failure to elicit peristalsis with distention is greater than that after swallowing.

In addition to the primary peristaltic wave, phasic, nonpropulsive contractions can be seen in the lower esophagus. In the elderly these are common (43), and in asymptomatic young subjects they can also be seen (33).

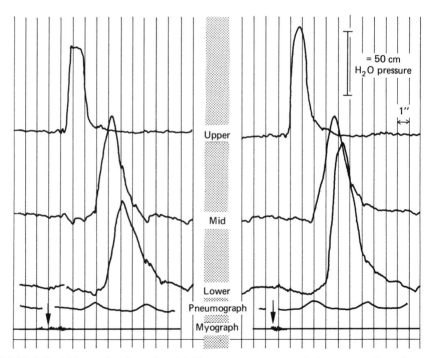

FIGURE 11-2.   Esophageal peristaltic pressure sequence during consecutive "dry" swallows in a healthy person. (From C. F. Code et al.: *An Atlas of Esophageal Motility in Health and Disease.* Springfield, Ill.: Charles C Thomas, Publisher, 1958.)

Upper Esophageal Sphincter

At the level of the cricopharyngeus, a high-pressure zone of about 39 cm H_2O extends over a width of 3 cm (16). With swallowing, the pressure promptly falls to near zero and then rises again rapidly to normal levels (2). One individual was studied who could relax his sphincter at will without swallowing.

Lower Esophageal Sphincter

Many investigators have described an area at the distal end of the esophagus that does not participate in the primary peristaltic wave. After swallowing, this zone showed a fall in pressure (14,17,26,38,45). Fyke et al. reported a high-pressure zone (10.7 cm H_2O above that in the stomach) extending 1 to 2 cm above the diaphragm and 1 to 2 cm below the diaphragmatic hiatus. It was 3 cm in width (17). Within 1 to 2 seconds of swallowing, the pressure fell to zero and returned to normal as the primary peristaltic wave reached the area. Using a layered column of radiopaque liquid, Fleshler et al. found that the sphincter mechanism resisted a force of 9 to 13 mm Hg (14). In healthy young subjects the pressures in this area were more variable than in the upper esophageal sphincter (33,34). In the aged, the fall in pressure in response to swallowing was frequently absent (43). In infants, regurgitation of barium from stomach to esophagus occurred freely in 46 per cent (4). Pressure studies showed poor development of resistance at the esophagogastric junction up to six days of life, then a gradual increase up to one year (18).

As noted earlier there is no agreement on the anatomic basis for the lower esophageal sphincter mechanism. In most reports the physiologic evidence places the sphincter at or above the diaphragmatic hiatus. During manometric studies, the direction of the phasic change in pressure coincident with respiration changes. Below the diaphragm, it falls with expiration and rises with inspiration, while above the diaphragm the response is reversed. Harris and Pope found that the site of reversal was more closely related to the sphincter than to the location of the diaphragm (21).

Harris and his associates have also raised the question of the significance of measuring contraction or "squeeze" as opposed to the resistance to distention (19,35,48). By adding a small catheter through which a very slow infusion of saline was pumped, they showed that the resistance to distention correlated much better with gastroesophageal reflux than the level of resting pressure.

Electrical Properties of Smooth Muscle of Esophagus

Longitudinal smooth muscle from the esophagus of cats showed only a few contractions at rest, and electrical slow waves as found elsewhere in intestinal longitudinal smooth muscle were rarely seen (7). When contractions were induced, bursts of spike potentials occurred accompanied by slow waves. In dogs, there was no electrical counterpart to relaxation of the lower esophageal sphincter, but in monkeys inhibition of electrical activity occurred prior to contraction (22,23).

Swallowing

It is customary to divide deglutition into oral, pharyngeal, and esophageal phases. However, the act of swallowing is so well coordinated that such a division becomes arbitrary. Most of our knowledge of the events during swallowing come from cineradiographic studies or from the observation of the rare patient whose surgical care exposes the structures of the pharynx to view. A simplification of events may be summarized by noting that the tongue, in contact with the hard palate, propels the food bolus into the pharynx at a time when the nasopharynx is closed by the soft palate and the airway is protected by closure of the glottis and tipping of the epiglottis in such a fashion as to divert material away from the glottis (36,37). The constrictor muscles of the pharynx propel the bolus into the esophagus. A negative pressure wave in the upper esophagus was recorded in one third of swallowing complexes and coincided with a falling intrapleural pressure (47). During swallowing the larynx rises and the pharynx is also elevated (44).

Control of Esophageal Motor Function

In general, cholinergic stimuli cause contraction of the tubular esophagus and relaxation of the lower esophageal sphincter (8). However, epinephrine caused contraction of the intact esophagus in the cat and similarly of circular muscle at the gastroesophageal junction (9,39). Acetylcholine relaxed the cardiac sphincter in the cat but atropine had little effect. In man, epinephrine and norepinephrine as well as adrenergic blockers had no effect on the function of the cardia (42). Below the upper third of the esophagus, atropine prolonged the duration of the swallowing complexes (28).

Swallowing itself is under the control of the central nervous system. Normally swallowing is initiated by stimulation of afferent nerves in the oropharynx. In man, the optimum sites for stimulation are on the anterior pillars (5). The efferent pathway involves the vagus, but Hwang and Grossman were unable to elicit swallowing by stimulation of nerves around the larynx in cadavers (24). In the rat, Andrew recorded electrical activity in both afferent and efferent fibers during swallowing. He found two types of efferent neurons—one to the upper esophagus, which exhibited tonic activity, and one responsible for peristalsis. The fibers concerned with tonic activity showed an interruption during swallowing, making them good candidates for supplying the upper esophageal sphincter. He also detected stretch receptors which might participate in the secondary peristaltic response (1).

The extrinsic nerves are involved in swallowing, as demonstrated by the persistence of the peristaltic waves after transection of the esophagus in dogs (40) and man (29). Swallowing movements can be elicited by stimulation of the cerebral cortex (5), but the major portion of the control system lies in the medullary reticular formation. Human monsters having no normal neural tissue rostral to the red nucleus can still swallow normally (13). In experimental animals, swallowing activity remains normal as long as the brain is intact from the level of the motor nucleus of the fifth cranial nerve.

As far as can be determined, the pathways in the central nervous system are similar for primary and secondary peristalsis (15,25,40). With repeated swallows, primary peristalsis is inhibited until after the last swallow (38).

Function of the Esophagus in Man

The esophagus in man consists of a hollow tube with a distinct muscular sphincter at the upper end and a complex arrangement involving the diaphragm, phrenoesophageal ligament, and stomach at the lower end, which functions as a sphincter. During swallowing, the upper sphincter relaxes first, followed by a peristaltic wave in the tubular portion of the esophagus and relaxation of the lower sphincter mechanism. A similar peristaltic contraction can be elicited by distention of the body of the esophagus. Swallowing is under the control of the central nervous system, and in particular afferent and efferent connections meet in a swallowing "center" in the medulla.

Pathophysiology

The measurement of pressures within the esophagus, or esophageal manometry, has become an investigative tool and subspecialized diagnostic service in gastroenterology. Disordered swallowing may occur in diseases involving the central nervous organization of deglutition, such as midbrain strokes, or peripheral neurons, as in poliomyelitis. Muscular diseases such as myasthenia gravis may present with weakened swallowing mechanisms. Pharyngeal diverticula may interfere with normal swallowing. The primary peristaltic wave is reduced in scleroderma involving the body of the esophagus, and disorders of the distal sphincter may lead to dysphagia, as in achalasia or esophagitis secondary to gastric reflux in hiatal hernia (12a). Harris wrote that manometry was of greatest value in the study of achalasia, diffuse spasm, and scleroderma (20). Achalasia is characterized by a failure of the lower esophageal sphincter to relax, with resulting obstruction. Histologic examination of the lower esophagus showed an absence of ganglion cells. Administration of a parasympathomimetic drug elicits a marked contraction, possibly a manifestation of the phenomenon of sensitization to the neurohumor by denervation. Diffuse spasm is a motor disorder in which the peristaltic activity is replaced by phasic contractions occurring simultaneously over the esophagus.

Acute esophageal obstruction produces not only secondary peristalsis but also a sustained contraction at the site of obstruction of great force (49). Certainly from the point of view of numbers, hiatal hernia represents an important clinical problem. The use of anticholinergics in this disease balances the reduction of gastric acid secretion against weakening of the sphincter mechanism (41). It is of interest that belching is associated with relaxation of the esophagogastric junction (30).

References

1. Andrew, B. L. The nervous control of the cervical oesophagus of the rat during swallowing. *J. Physiol. London* **134:** 729–740, 1956.
2. Atkinson, M., P. Kramer, S. M. Wyman, and F. J. Inglefinger. The dynamics of swallowing. I. Normal pharyngeal mechanisms. *J. Clin. Invest.* **36:** 581–588, 1957.
3. Atkinson, M. Mechanisms protecting against gastro-oesophageal reflux: A review. *Gut* **3:** 1–15, 1962.
4. Blank, L., and W. L. Pew. Cardio-esophageal relaxation (chalasia) studies on the normal infant. *Am. J. Roentgenol.* **76:** 540–550, 1956.
5. Bosma, J. F. Deglutition: Pharyngeal stage. *Physiol. Rev.* **37:** 275–300, 1957.
6. Butin, J. W., A. M. Olsen, H. J. Moersch, and C. F. Code. A study of esophageal pressure in normal persons and patients with cardiospasm. *Gastroenterology* **23:** 278–291, 1953.
7. Christensen, J., and E. E. Daniel. Electric and motor effects of autonomic drugs on longitudinal esophageal smooth muscle. *Am. J. Physiol.* **211:** 387–394, 1966.
8. Christensen, J. Pharmacology of the esophagus. In: *Handbook of Physiology.* Section 6: Alimentary Tract. Vol. IV: Motility. Edited by C. F. Code. Washington, D.C.: American Physiological Society, 1968. pp. 2325–2330.
9. Clark, C. G., and J. R. Vane. The cardiac sphincter in the cat. *Gut* **2:** 252–262, 1961.
10. Code, C. F., B. Creamer, J. F. Schlegel, A. M. Olsen, F. E. Donoghue, and H. A. Anderson. *An Atlas of Esophageal Motility in Health and Disease.* Springfield, Ill.: Charles C Thomas, 1958.
11. Code, C. F., and J. F. Schlegel. Motor action of the esophagus and its sphincters. In *Handbook of Physiology.* Section 6: Alimentary Tract. Vol. IV: Motility. Edited by C. F. Code. Washington, D.C.: American Physiological Society, 1968, pp. 1821–1839.
12. Cohen, B. R., and B. S. Wolf. Cineradiographic and intraluminal pressure correlations in the pharynx and esophagus. In: *Handbook of Physiology.* Section 6: Alimentary Tract. Vol. IV: Motility. Edited by C. F. Code. Washington, D.C.: American Physiological Society, 1968, pp. 1841–1860.

12a Creamer, B. Motor disturbances of the esophagus. In: *Handbook of Physiology*. Section 6: Alimentary Tract. Vol. IV: Motility. Edited by C. F. Code. Washington, D.C.: American Physiological Society, 1968, pp. 2331–2343.

13. Doty, R. W. Neural organization of deglutition. In: *Handbook of Physiology*. Section 6: Alimentary Tract. Vol. IV: Motility. Edited by C. F. Code. Washington, D.C.: American Physiological Society, 1968, pp. 1861–1902.

14. Fleshler, B., T. R. Hendrix, P. Kramer, and F. J. Inglefinger. Resistance and reflex function of the lower esophageal sphincter. *J. Appl. Physiol.* **12:** 339–342, 1958.

15. Fleshler, B., T. R. Hendrix, P. Kramer, and F. J. Inglefinger. The characteristics and similarity of primary and secondary peristalsis in the esophagus. *J. Clin. Invest.* **38:** 110–116, 1959.

16. Fyke, F. E., Jr., and C. F. Code. Resting and deglutition pressures in the pharyngoesophageal region. *Gastroenterology* **29:** 24–34, 1955.

17. Fyke, F. E., Jr., C. F. Code, and J. F. Schlegel. The gastroesophageal sphincter in healthy human beings. *Gastroenterologia* **86:** 135–150, 1956.

18. Gryboski, J. D., W. R. Thayer, Jr., and H. M. Spiro. Esophageal motility in infants and children. *Pediatrics* **31:** 382–395, 1963.

19. Harris, L. D., and C. E. Pope, II. "Squeeze" vs. resistance: An evaluation of the mechanism of sphincter competence. *J. Clin. Invest.* **43:** 2272–2278, 1964.

20. Harris, L. D. Present status of esophageal manometry. *Gastroenterology* **50:** 708–710, 1966.

21. Harris, L. D., and C. E. Pope, II. The pressure inversion point; its genesis and reliability. *Gastroenterology* **51:** 641–648, 1966.

22. Hellemans, J., and G. Vantrappen. Electromyographic studies on canine esophageal motility. *Am. J. Dig. Dis.* **12:** 1240–1255, 1967.

23. Hellemans, G., G. Vantrappen, P. Valembois, J. Janssens, and J. Vandenbroucke. Electrical activity of striated and smooth muscle of the esophagus. *Am. J. Dig. Dis.* **13:** 320–334, 1968.

24. Hwang, K., and M. I. Grossman. A note on the innervation of the cervical portion of the human esophagus. *Gastroenterology* **25:** 375–377, 1953.

25. Hwang, K. Mechanism of transportation of the content of the esophagus. *J. Appl. Physiol.* **6:** 781–796, 1954.

26. Inglefinger, F. J., P. Kramer, and G. C. Sanchez. The gastro-esophageal vestibule; its normal function and its role in cardiospasm and gastroesophageal reflux. *Am. J. Med. Sci.* **228:** 417–425, 1954.

27. Inglefinger, F. J. Esophageal motility. *Physiol. Rev.* **38:** 533–584, 1958.

28. Kantrowitz, P. A., C. I. Siegel, and T. R. Hendrix. Differences in motility of the upper and lower esophagus in man and its alterations by atropine. *Bull. Johns Hopkins Hosp.* **118:** 476–491, 1966.

29. Kramer, P. Esophagus. *Gastroenterology* **54:** 1171–1192, 1968.

30. McNally, E. F., J. E. Kelly, Jr., and F. J. Inglefinger. Mechanism of belching: Effects of gastric distention with air. *Gastroenterology* **46:** 254–259, 1964.

31. Meckeler, K. J. H., and F. J. Inglefinger. Correlation of electric surface potentials, intraluminal pressures, and nature of tissue in the gastroesophageal junction of man. *Gastroenterology* **52:** 966–971, 1967.

32. Michelson, E., and C. I. Siegel. The role of the phrenicoesophageal ligament in the lower esophageal sphincter. *Surg. Gynce. Obstet.* **118:** 1291–1294, 1964.

33. Nagler, R., and H. M. Spiro. Serial esophageal motility studies in asymptomatic young subjects. *Gastroenterology* **41:** 371–379, 1961.

34. Pert, J. H., M. Davidson, T. P. Almy, and M. H. Sleisenger. Esophageal catheterization studies. I. The mechanism of swallowing in normal subjects with particular reference to the vestibule (esophago-gastric sphincter). *J. Clin. Invest.* **38:** 397–406, 1959.

35. Pope, C. E., II. A dynamic test of sphincter strength: Its application to the lower esophageal sphincter. *Gastroenterology* **52:** 779–786, 1967.

36. Ramsey, G. H., J. S. Watson, R. Gramiak, and S. A. Weinberg. Cinefluorographic analysis of the mechanism of swallowing. *Radiology* **64:** 498–518, 1955.

37. Rushmer, R. F., and J. A. Hendron. The act of deglutition. A cinefluorographic study. *J. Appl. Physiol.* **3:** 622–630, 1951.

38. Sanchez, G. C., P. Kramer, and F. J. Inglefinger. Motor mechanisms of the esophagus, particularly of its distal portion. *Gastroenterology* **25:** 321–332, 1953.

39. Schenk, E. A., and E. L. Frederickson. Pharmacologic evidence for a cardiac sphincter mechanism in the cat. *Gastroenterology* **40:** 75–80, 1961.

40. Siegel, C. I., and T. R. Hendrix. Evidence for central mediation of secondary peristalsis in esophagus. *Bull. Johns Hopkins Hosp.* **108:** 297–307, 1961.

41. Skinner, D. B., and T. F. Camp, Jr. Relation of esophageal reflux to lower esophageal sphincter pressures decreased by atropine. *Gastroenterology* **54:** 543–551, 1968.

42. Sleisenger, M. H., H. Steinberg, and T. P. Almy. The disturbance of esophageal motility in cardiospasm: Studies on autonomic stimulation and autonomic blockade of the human esophagus including the cardia. *Gastroenterology* **25:** 333–348, 1953.

43. Soergel, K. H., F. F. Zboralske, and J. R. Amberg. Presbyesophagus: Esophageal motility in nonagenarians. *J. Clin. Invest.* **43:** 1472–1479, 1964.

44. Sokol, E. M., P. Heitmann, B. S. Wolf, and B. R. Cohen. Simultaneous cineradiographic and manometric study of the pharynx, hypopharynx, and cervical esophagus. *Gastroenterology* **51:** 960–974, 1966.

45. Texter, E. C., H. W. Smith, H. C. Moeller, and C. J. Baborka. Intraluminal pressures from the upper gastrointestinal tract. I. Correlations with motor activity in normal subjects and patients with esophageal disorders. *Gastroenterology* **32:** 1013–1024, 1957.

46. Van Derstappen, G., and E. C. Texter Jr. Response of the physiologic gastroesophageal sphincter to increased intra-abdominal pressure. *J. Clin. Invest.* **43:** 1856–1868, 1964.

47. Vantrappen, G., and J. Hellemans. Studies on the normal deglutition complex. *Am. J. Dig. Dis.* **12:** 255–266, 1967.

48. Winans, C. S., and L. D. Harris. Quantitation of lower esophageal sphincter competence. *Gastroenterology* **52:** 773–778, 1967.

49. Winship, D. H., and F. F. Zboralske. The esophageal propulsive force: Esophageal response to acute obstruction. *J. Clin. Invest.* **46:** 1391–1401, 1967.

50. Wolf, B. S., R. H. Marshak, M. L. Som, S. A. Brahms, and E. I. Greenberg. The gastroesophageal vestibule on roentgen examination: Differentiation from the phrenic ampulla and minimal hiatal herniation. *J. Mt. Sinai Hosp. N.Y.* **25:** 167–200, 1958.

51. Wolf, B. S. Roentgen features of the normal and herniated esophagogastric region. *Am. J. Dig. Dis.* **5:** 751–769, 1960.

CHAPTER

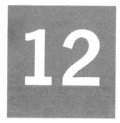

Gastric Motility and Emptying

THE MOTOR FUNCTION OF THE STOMACH is concerned with mixing and grinding the gastric content and finally delivering it into the duodenum at an appropriate rate. Following partial removal of the stomach in man, the most troublesome symptoms result from a loss of the reservoir function of the stomach and the resulting rapid emptying of gastric content incompletely prepared into the small intestine.

From the point of view of its motor function the stomach can be divided into three portions—the cardiac portion or fundus, lying above the level of the entrance of the esophagus; the body; and the pyloric antrum. The cardiac region is concerned with adapting to the entrance of food. The body of the stomach serves as a vat where the food is acted upon by acid-pepsin, and the pyloric antrum acts as a grinding mill. Pouches of the cardiac region in dogs show most commonly a slow phasic change in pressure. These were present about 80 per cent of the time the pouch was active and lasted one to two minutes. Recorded with small balloons, the amplitude measured 10 to 25 cm of water. Following swallows, inhibition of motor activity and reduction of pressure in the pouch occurred 57 per cent of the time. This probably represents the phenomenon of receptive relaxation (21).

The characterization of the motor activity of the body and pyloric antrum will depend very much on the techniques of study. Historically balloons were used to record gastric contractions, usually of such a size that the activity of the body and the antrum were recorded simultaneously. Later open-tipped catheters were used. Misinterpretations occurred because of the ability of the stomach to divide itself into a series of closed chambers. Radiographic cine-

168

matography gave a dynamic picture of pyloric activity but gave no information about pressure. More recently telemetering pressure sensors or "radio pills" have been used but are difficult to keep in a particular portion of the stomach. Code and Carlson advocate a classification of gastric contractile activity based upon functional significance (9). They define four types of activity—tonic contractions, peristaltic contractions, terminal antral contractions, and fundic waves. Tonic contractions have the function of diminishing the capacity of the segment of stomach involved. They include the contractions in the fundus already described and in the pyloric antrum. In man, after an overnight fast, they can be recorded about 10 to 30 per cent of the time during the first two hours from the antral region (9). Their occurrence is not altered by meals or by distention of the antrum. The pressures produced in balloons by tonic antral contractions in man range between 2 and 5 cm of water. Their mean duration was 53 seconds. They may have an important function in the antrum by altering the output of the antral pump.

Peristaltic contractions result from contraction of a band of circular muscle fibers surrounding the stomach which moves caudally as a result of progressive contraction and relaxation of fibers. The advancing face consists of contracting fibers, while at the distal face, relaxation occurs. The width of the band is about 1 to 2 cm. Radiographic studies indicate that the contractions begin high on the lesser curvature and sweep distally to the pylorus. Some contractions gradually cease in the antrum, some pass with increasing vigor to end at the pylorus, and some end with simultaneous contractions of the terminal antrum and pyloric canal. The vigorous contractions continuing into the antrum are usually associated with emptying of the stomach (31), while those that fade out are not. The latter have an amplitude of 5 cm when recorded with balloons of 3-cm diameter. The former contractions usually exceed 5 cm, in amplitude but the distinction is arbitrary. In man, the maximum frequency of contractions is 3 per minute, denoted as 20-second rhythm by Carlson. They may or may not occur in rhythmic fashion. Peristaltic waves serve two functions—mixing of gastric content and, for those of larger amplitude, emptying of the stomach. The mixing activity is present for the greater proportion of the day.

Terminal antral contractions involve the last 4 to 5 cm of the antrum and the pyloric canal. Terminal antral contraction and contraction that closes the pyloric canal start simultaneously. Since the canal is narrow, it usually empties and closes earlier than the antrum and remains closed throughout the remainder of the terminal antral contraction. The frequency of the terminal antral contractions follows that of peristaltic contractions. They serve the function of mixing, reducing the size of particles, and emulsifying gastric contents. When the pyloric canal closes, the antral contents are expelled in a retrograde fashion into the body of the stomach. The proximal end of the antrum is usually narrowed at the time by the peristaltic contraction so that there is a nozzle effect which contributes to the mixing. There is also a rubbing and grinding effect. Motor activity is present more often in the antrum than elsewhere in the stomach. High pressures when the antrum is compressed between closure of the pylorus and an advancing peristaltic contraction can be shown in the stomach in vitro during transmural electrical stimulation (3).

Open-tipped catheters in the body of the stomach would fail to record contractions of the antrum under these circumstances. The same would obtain with telemetering pressure sensors. Silverstone et al. found a reasonably good correlation between pressure sensors and catheters in man, but about 20 per cent of large-amplitude peristaltic contractions were recorded by one and not the other (30). In dogs, force transducers can be sutured to longitudinal or circular muscle layers. The maximal contractile force occurred in the circular muscle, but the force in both longitudinal and circular muscle in the stomach was greater than that in the intestine. The velocity of contraction was greater in the antrum and in longitudinal muscle compared to circular (29).

In the fasting stomach, contractions may increase in amplitude and be recognized by the human subject as "hunger pangs." It has become fashionable to deprecate any role of these contractions in the sensation of hunger, in part because gastrectomized subjects still experience "hunger." Code and Carlson advocate use of the term *prandial contractions* (9). However, the original correlations have never been disproved and indeed recent studies indicate that subjects can be taught to recognize contractions of the stomach coincident with hunger with a high degree of accuracy (15). Following eating, large-amplitude peristaltic contractions decrease in frequency, although small-amplitude contractions may remain unchanged (32). After a breakfast containing 16 gm of fat, normal subjects showed an increase in total activity during the second hour. With a breakfast containing 100 gm of fat, large-amplitude peristaltic contractions were abolished. In dogs, with force transducers, bursts of activity occurred during the interdigestive period but were abolished after eating (27). During digestion, higher amplitude contractions occurred in the antrum than in the body (1).

Control of Gastric Contractions

The vagus nerves occupy a central role in the control of gastric contractions. Martinson found two populations of efferent nerve fibers in the vagi of anesthetized cats. One group was characterized by low thresholds to electrical stimulation and produced excitation. The other was composed of high-threshold fibers and upon stimulation led to inhibition of contractile activity (24). In conscious dogs, using different recording techniques, two groups of investigators found that sham feeding reduced the frequency of large-amplitude peristaltic contractions (22,26). Unfortunately in neither experiment was the role of acid secretion entering the intestine defined, but insulin-hypoglycemia in the same animals stimulated peristaltic contractions (26).

Two other vagal stimulants, 2-deoxyglucose and insulin, excite peristaltic contractions. Insulin produced inhibition followed by excitation in dogs with innervated antral pouches, while the effect of 2-deoxyglucose was more variable (20,35). Grahame et al., using dogs with gastric fistulas, found that 2-deoxyglucose increased contractions and pepsin secretion in parallel while histamine stimulated only secretion of acid (14). Stimulation of the hypothalamus and amygdala produced inhibition of gastric contractions in conscious dogs which was abolished by vagotomy (12). It should be noted that Martinson considered the chemical transmitter in vagal inhibitory efferents to be unknown.

There is a large volume of literature implicating humoral factors in the control of gastric contractions. Secretin and cholecystokinin-pancreozymin have been suspected to be inhibitors. The ability to obtain single molecular species should help define their role, but the problem of physiologic significance remains. The interpretation of the effect of extracts is very difficult (6,7,18,19). The existence of a blood-borne inhibitor of gastric contractions following fat in the duodenum seems clear, but the chemical nature of "enterogastrone" is still unknown (34).

Recent studies show that gastrin has a selective excitatory effect on the stomach, both in vitro and in vivo (5,25). Vagal stimulation in vitro liberated prostaglandin E from rat stomach, possibly by distorting the cells producing the substance (4,8).

In man, vagotomy is followed by a decrease in both the resting intraluminal pressure and the number of contractions. After a few months, however, contractile activity returns toward normal (34). The effects of the sympathetic division of the autonomic nervous system are less well known. Thoracolumbar sympathectomy had little effect on gastric motor function in man.

The effects of stimulation of autonomic nerve fibers on contractions of the gastrointestinal tract in anesthetized animals can be conflicting (38). Most of the effects involve the contraction or relaxation of the muscularis propria, and the function of the muscularis mucosae has been neglected. Walder found that acetylcholine applied to this tissue in vitro always elicited contraction, whereas epinephrine produced variable results depending upon the source of the muscle. The latter caused contractions of strips from the greater curvature but relaxation of those from the lesser curve (37). Since hexamethonium blocked both contraction and relaxation, he concluded that ganglion cells in the submucosal plexus included both cholinergic and adrenergic neurons.

Acid in Heidenhain pouches, if it can penetrate the mucosal barrier, stimulates gastric contractions (10). Acetic acid was effective, but hydrochloric acid succeeded only if the barrier was broken.

Gastric Emptying

The emptying of the stomach serves as a quantitative function for assessing the motor activity of the stomach as a whole. As a result of the studies of

Thomas and Quigley, emptying of the stomach was considered to be the result of a pressure gradient between the stomach and the duodenum. In the resting state, the basal antral pressure is only 1 to 2 cm of water greater than that in the duodenum. As peristaltic contractions spread over the antrum, the pressure rises to 15 to 30 cm of water. The pressure in the duodenum also rises, and both may reach a peak at about the same time. A pressure gradient of 2 to 30 cm of water may exist during the later phase of gastric contraction when emptying occurs. Rhodes et al. found that a fall in duodenal pH occurred coincident with antral contractions in man (28).

The time course of gastric emptying can be determined by the use of test meals. A fixed volume of meal was given to subjects on repeated occasions, and the stomach emptied at a different time after the meal on each occasion. This permitted a plot of the amount of material remaining in the stomach at different times. Incorporating an inert marker into the meal permitted the determination of the degree of dilution of the contents by gastric secretion. The data presented in Figures 12-1 and 12-2 illustrate the results. It can be seen that emptying occurs more rapidly early after the meal than later (16). More recently George has modified the procedure to permit sampling at repeated intervals after a single meal (13).

Various factors effect emptying of the stomach. Larger volumes accelerate emptying, and meals with larger food particles empty more slowly. Carbohydrates, proteins, and fat leave the stomach in increasing order.

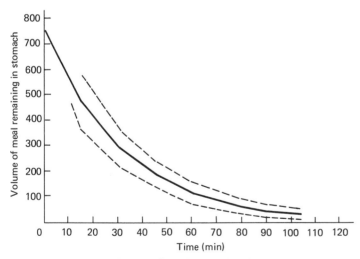

FIGURE 12-1.   Volume of meal remaining in stomach plotted against time. (19 subjects.) ---, weighted mean; . . . . , standard deviation. (From J. N. Hunt. J. Physiol. London 113: 157–168, 1951.)

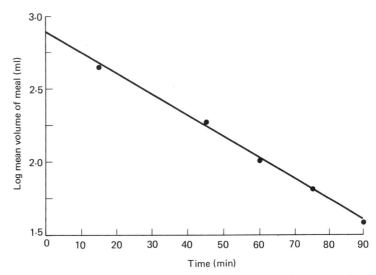

FIGURE 12-2.   Log mean volume of meal remaining in the stomach plotted against time in 19 subjects including points from 15 to 90 minutes. (From J. N. Hunt. *J. Physiol. London* **113:** 157–168, 1951.)

Control of Gastric Emptying

Distention of the stomach to a modest degree is the only physiologic mechanism known to act on the stomach to accelerate gastric emptying. Delay of gastric emptying seems to depend largely upon duodenal factors. Hunt has emphasized the role of hypothetical osmoreceptors in the duodenum in the control of gastric emptying (*16*). He based his suggestion on the observation of the differences between solutes that penetrate cell membranes and those that penetrate slowly or not at all. He suggested that the latter cause shrinking of the receptor cells and signal a delay in gastric emptying, presumably by reducing the contractile activity of the stomach.

Fatty acids with twelve or more carbon atoms reduce emptying in proportion to their molecular size (*17*). It was not possible to determine whether the same osmoreceptor responds to acid, carbohydrate, and fat or to only one. Thomas doubts that amino acids and fats act entirely by an effect on osmoreceptors and points out that the evidence is entirely indirect (*34*). Since disaccharides seem to effect gastric emptying after hydrolysis to monosaccharides, Hunt has suggested that the osmoreceptors must lie deep to the brush border (*11*).

The action of fat in delaying gastric emptying remains something of an enigma. Hunt, on the basis of the time course of inhibition by repeated injections of fat, doubted that a hormonal mechanism was operating in man. Bilateral vagotomy depressed the delaying effect of fat after gastroenterostomy (36). Recently Anderson et al., using duodenal pouches, found no effect of fat in the pouch on contractile force in the stomach (2). Despite the controversy over the mechanism, fat remains the best dietary means for delaying gastric emptying.

Other factors affecting gastric emptying include substances binding calcium such as oxalate (33) and saliva in man (23).

Pathophysiology

Vagotomy alone is an unsatisfactory procedure in the treatment of duodenal ulcer because it produced gastric stasis. Anticholinergic drugs may convert a partially obstructed stomach into complete obstruction. Fats, by delaying gastric emptying, may facilitate neutralization of gastric acid in the treatment of ulcer. Following gastric resection and gastrojejunal anastomosis, swallowed liquid passes quickly into the jejunum. If the solution is hypertonic, fluid is drawn into the jejunum, the wall is distended, and the plasma volume falls. With these phenomena, the patient experiences weakness, flushing, and lightheadedness—the symptoms of the dumping syndrome.

References

1. Anderson, J. J., R. J. Bolt, B. M. Ullman, and P. Bass. Differential response to various stimulants in the body and antrum of the canine stomach. *Am. J. Dig. Dis.* **13**: 147–156, 1968.
2. Anderson, J. J., R. J. Bolt, B. M. Ullman, and P. Bass. Effect of bile and fat on gastric motility under the influence of various stimulants. *Am. J. Dig. Dis.* **13**: 157–167, 1968.
3. Armitage, A. K., and A. C. B. Dean. Function of the pylorus and pyloric antrum in gastric emptying. *Gut* **4**: 174–178, 1963.
4. Bennett, A., C. A. Friedmann, and J. R. Vane. Release of prostaglandin E_1 from the rat stomach. *Nature* **216**: 873–876, 1967.
5. Bennett, A., J. J. Misiewicz, and S. L. Waller. Analysis of the motor effects of gastrin and pentagastrin on the human alimentary tract in vitro. *Gut* **8**: 470–474, 1967.
6. Brown, J. C. Presence of a gastric-motor-stimulating property in duodenal extracts. *Gastroenterology* **52**: 225–229, 1967.
7. Brown, J. C., and C. O. Parkes. Effect on fundic pouch motor activity of stimulatory and inhibitory fractions separated from pancreozymin. *Gastroenterology* **53**: 731–736, 1967.
8. Cocea, F., C. Pace-Asciak, F. Volta, and L. S. Wolfe. Effect of nerve stimulation on prostaglandin formation and release from the rat stomach. *Am. J. Physiol.* **213**: 1056–1064, 1967.

9. Code, C. F., and H. C. Carlson. Motor activity of the stomach. In: *Handbook of Physiology*. Section 6: Alimentary Tract. Vol. IV: Motility. Edited by C. F. Code. Washington, D.C.: American Physiological Society, 1968, pp. 1903–1916.

10. Davenport, H. W. Stimulation of gastric motility by acid. *Gastroenterology* 52: 198–204, 1967.

11. Elias, E., G. J. Gibson, L. F. Greenwood, J. N. Hunt, and J. H. Tripp. The slowing of gastric emptying by monosaccharides and disaccharides in test meals. *J. Physiol. London* 194: 317–326, 1968.

12. Fennegan, F. M., and M. J. Puiggari. Hypothalamic and amygdaloid influence on gastric motility in dogs. *J. Neurosurg.* 24: 497–504, 1966.

13. George, J. D. New clinical method for measuring the rate of gastric emptying: The double sampling test meal. *Gut* 9: 237–242, 1968.

14. Grahame, G. R., J. M. Garrett, and B. I. Hirschowitz. 2-Deoxyglucose and histamine effects on gastric motility and secretion in the dog. *Am. J. Physiol.* 215: 243–248, 1968.

15. Griggs, R. C., and A. Stunkard. The interpretation of gastric motility. *Arch. Gen. Psychiat.* 11: 82–89, 1964.

16. Hunt, J. N., and M. T. Knox. Regulation of gastric emptying. In: *Handbook of Physiology*. Section 6: Alimentary Tract. Vol. IV: Motility. Edited by C. F. Code. Washington, D.C.: American Physiological Society, pp. 1917–1935.

17. Hunt, J. N., and M. T. Knox. A relation between the chain length of fatty acids and the slowing of gastric emptying. *J. Physiol. London* 194: 327–336, 1968.

18. Johnson, L. P., and D. F. Magee. Cholecystokinin-pancreozymin extracts and gastric motor inhibition. *Surg. Gynec. Obstet.* 121: 557–562, 1965.

19. Johnson, L. P., J. C. Brown, and D. F. Magee. Effect of secretin and cholecystokinin-pancreozymin extracts on gastric motility in man. *Gut* 7: 52–57, 1966.

20. Kemp, D. R., R. Herrera, M. Tsukamoto, and M. M. Eisenberg. Insulin-potassium effect on gastric acid secretion and antral motility in dogs. *Gastroenterology* 54: 190–196, 1968.

21. Lind, J. F., H. L. Duthie, J. F. Schlegel, and C. F. Code. Motility of the gastric fundus. *Am. J. Physiol.* 201: 197–202, 1961.

22. Lorber, S. H., S. A. Komarov, and H. Shay. Effect of sham feeding on gastric motor activity of the dog. *Am. J. Physiol.* 162: 447–451, 1950.

23. Malhotra, S. L. Effect of saliva on gastric emptying. *Am. J. Physiol.* 213: 169–173, 1967.

24. Martinson, J. Studies on the efferent control of the stomach. *Acta Physiol. Scand.* 65: Suppl. 255: 1–24, 1965.

25. Misiewicz, J. J., D. J. Holdstock, and S. L. Waller. Motor responses of the human alimentary tract to near-maximal infusions of pentagastrin. *Gut* 8: 463–469, 1967.

26. Olbe, L., and B. Jacobson. Intraluminal pressure waves of the stomach in dogs studied by radiosondes. *Gastroenterology* 44: 787–796, 1963.

27. Reinke, D. A., A. H. Rosenbaum, and D. R. Bennett. Patterns of dog gastrointestinal contractile activity monitored in vivo with extraluminal force transducers. *Am. J. Dig. Dis.* 12: 113–141, 1967.

28. Rhodes, J., P. Goodall, and H. T. Apsimon. Mechanics of gastroduodenal emptying. *Gut* 7: 515–520, 1966.

29. Rosenbaum, A. H., D. A. Reinke, and D. R. Bennett. In-vivo force frequency

and velocity of dog gastrointestinal contractile activity. *Am. J. Dig. Dis.* **12:** 142–153, 1967.

30. Silverstone, J. T., G. P. Smith, and A. J. Stunkard. Gastric pressures recorded by a telemetering capsule. *Am. J. Dig. Dis.* **13:** 615–618, 1968.

31. Smith, A. W. M., C. F. Code, and J. F. Schlegel. Simultaneous cineradiographic and kymographic studies of human gastric antral motility. *J. Appl. Physiol.* **11:** 12–16, 1957

32. Smith, A. W. M., and C. F. Code. The effect of an ordinary and of an excessively fatty breakfast on human gastric antral motility. *Gastroenterology* **35:** 398–405, 1958.

33. Sognen, E. Effects of calcium-binding substances on gastric emptying as well as intestinal transit and absorption in intact rats. *Acta Pharmacol. (Kobenhavn)* **22:** 31–48, 1965.

34. Thomas, J. E., and M. V. Baldwin. Pathways and mechanisms of regulation of gastric motility. In: *Handbook of Physiology.* Section 6: Alimentary Tract. Vol. IV: Edited by C. F. Code. Washington, D.C.: American Physiological Society, 1968, pp. 1937–1968.

35. Tsukamoto, M., F. Herrera, D. R. Kemp, G. S. Emas, E. R. Woodward, and M. M. Eisenberg. Effect of vagal stimulation by 2-deoxy-D-glucose and insulin on gastric motility in dogs. *Ann. Surg.* **165:** 605–608, 1967.

36. Waddell, W. R., and C. C. Wang. The effect of vagotomy on gastric evacuation of high fat meals. *J. Appl. Physiol.* **5:** 705–711, 1953.

37. Walder, D. N. The muscularis mucosae of the human stomach. *J. Physiol. London* **120:** 365–372, 1953.

38. Youmans, W. B. Innervation of the gastrointestinal tract. In: *Handbook of Physiology.* Section 6: Alimentary Tract. Vol. IV: Motility. Edited by C. F. Code. Washington, D.C.: American Physiological Society, 1968, pp. 1655–1663.

Small Intestinal and Biliary Tract Motility

Small Intestinal Motility

The movement of the chyme into and through the small intestine is of considerable importance because of its effect on digestion and absorption. Mixing of the intestinal secretions with gastric content exposes the chyme to pancreatic enzymes and to bile, furthering the digestive process. Segmenting movements of the small intestine expose the intestinal mucosa to the digestion products for absorption. If transit through the intestine is too rapid to permit mixing and absorption, diarrhea and malabsorption may result. Under normal circumstances movement is adjusted nicely to permit nearly complete digestion and absorption.

STRUCTURAL BASIS FOR SMALL INTESTINAL MOTILITY

Smooth muscle is grouped in three layers—the muscularis mucosae, the circular muscle coat, and the longitudinal muscle coat (77). The myenteric plexus of Auerbach lies between the longitudinal and circular muscle layers, while the plexus of Meissner lies in the submucosa. Present concepts suggest that sympathetic adrenergic fibers synapse with ganglion cells in the myenteric plexuses which are also supplied by parasympathetic cholinergic neurons. Relatively few adrenergic fibers can be traced directly to smooth muscle. Unfortunately it is not possible to distinguish afferent from efferent fibers in the myenteric and submucosal plexuses, so that the exact nature of the organization of these neurons is unknown.

MOTILITY OF ISOLATED SEGMENTS OF INTESTINE

The ability of segments of intestine to contract in vitro led many workers to attempt a more specific analysis of intestinal movements in this preparation. A favorite experiment involves the ileum of the guinea pig, mounted in such a way that both a change in length and the volume of fluid in the lumen can be recorded. This permits an assessment of the function of the longitudinal and circular muscles. In response to distention, the segment shortens and expels its contents (63). By the use of pharmacologic agents and varying the degree of distention, the action of the longitudinal and circular muscles can be dissociated. The first phase of contraction of longitudinal muscle shows a graded response acting directly on the muscle. The emptying or peristaltic phase involves a cholinergic ganglion. The neurohumoral agent acting on the muscle in both phases is thought to be acetylcholine. The site of the receptor responding to distention is still debated (53). Various drugs modify the peristaltic reflex (14). While it has been an interesting system, the peculiarities of the guinea pig ileum limit the application of results to other animals.

AFFERENT FIBERS FROM THE INTESTINE

The features of afferent fibers in the vagi carrying sensory information from the intestine have already been noted. Some respond both to distention and to normal contractions. Recently afferents in the mesenteric nerves of cat have been isolated which discharge in relation to propulsive motor contractions. Bassou and Perl suggest that these may be movement receptors (16).

TRANSIT THROUGH THE GASTROINTESTINAL TRACT

The overall motor function of the gut can be assessed by feeding a marker such as radioactive chromium. In 8 of 10 normal human subjects, the total recoverable dose was passed within 96 hours. A third and two thirds were recovered after 24 and 48 hours respectively (42). Such a method does not permit determination of the specific parts of the gastrointestinal tract where delays might occur. Lish et al. (64) devised a technique in rats that permitted localization within the gut and found that glucagon, catecholamines, and 5-hydroxytryptamine all delayed small intestinal transit. Insulin delayed transit for the first 15 minutes after a subcutaneous dose but then markedly accelerated transit (64). Brown bread passed through the human gut faster than white bread (66).

THE ROLE OF THE PYLORODUODENAL SEGMENT IN INTESTINAL TRANSIT

The muscular thickening at the pylorus is an easily verified anatomic fact, yet when the pressure-sensing techniques described earlier were applied to the pylorus in man, there was no evidence of a sphincter mechanism (3,4). Only in dogs was a high-pressure zone of 3 to 11 cm of H_2O extending over a width of 1 to 2 cm demonstrated in 60 per cent of studies (17). The antrum and the pyloric ring behave like a single muscle mass (33). Cineradiographic studies in dogs showed two types of antral contractions, both starting near the cardia. One was a shallow ring with little propulsive effect. The other formed a deep contraction in the antrum. When it reached the terminal antrum, the entire segment contracted and forced the contents of the antrum back into the body of the stomach (19).

The relationship between motor activity in the antrum and duodenum is interesting, since the basic electrical rhythm of the stomach is about 3 or 4 slow waves per minute, while in the duodenum it is about 18 per minute. Allen et al. found no relation between the electrical slow waves at rest in dogs, but when the animals were fed, the spike activity in the duodenum bore a relation to the slow waves in the antrum (2).

Inhibitory mechanisms in the duodenum include the enterograstric reflex, which may be elicited by mechanical or chemical stimuli, and possible hormonal factors, secretin and enterogastrone. All result in a delay in gastric emptying (17,29).

Vagotomy reduced the inhibitory response to protein digestion products. Daniel suggested that the afferent limb of the enterogastric reflex may travel in the vagi and the efferent in the sympathetics (29).

MOTOR ACTIVITY OF THE SMALL INTESTINE

As in the stomach, the description of motor activity in the small intestine has been plagued with problems in methodology and terminology. Hightower suggested recently that contractions be defined as segmenting or peristaltic (49). Segmenting contractions are localized circumferential contractions involving primarily circular muscle. Peristaltic contractions are progressive but may be limited in distance and are not necessarily preceded by a wave of relaxation. Rhythmic contractions are unusual in the small gut, being present less than 2 per cent of the time (38).

Occasionally a patient may be available with a thin abdominal wall so that contractions of the intestine become visible through the wall. The most commonly present activity in such a patient was small constrictive rings traveling rapidly over a distance of a few centimeters. More foreceful contractions sometimes swept over an entire loop (41).

Motor activity has been studied intensively in terms of intraluminal pressures. Contractile activity was present about 60 to 70 per cent of the time after an overnight fast and less if the fast was prolonged (37). In the terminal ileum, Fink found activity 50 to 90 per cent of the time (35). Attempts to classify contractions on the basis of duration and amplitude have proven unsatisfactory (13,78). In infants and young children, activity was present 23 per cent of the time in the duodenum (6). Several groups of investigators have combined pressure studies with cineradiography. Deller and Wangel found that various wave forms could be propulsive at times but not at others. Progression of a contraction down the intestine did not guarantee propulsion (30). They concluded that an aboral pressure gradient was the most important factor in propulsion. Friedman and associates found monophasic waves in the duodenum measuring 2 to 40 mm Hg. Contractions superimposed on a rise in baseline were more common in the distal duodenum (38,39).

Telemetering pressure-sensing devices avoid the necessity for intubation. They can be tracked automatically. Feeding increased the number and amplitude of contractions. Propulsion also increased but could not be correlated with pressure signals (5). Phasic pressure rises superimposed on an increase in baseline were recorded rarely (50). Ramorino and Colagrande reported on simultaneous recordings from telemetering devices and cineradiography. They found that the contractions superimposed on a rise in tonus were usually propulsive (73). Farrar concluded that none of the available techniques permitted a functional classification of intestinal contractions (34).

Jacoby et al. described the implantation of force transducers into the longitudinal and circular muscle layers of intestinal muscles in dogs (54). They found that activity was at a low level in the fasting state with bursts of large-amplitude activity. After feeding, an intermediate type of activity predominated with very few bursts (74). There was no difference in maximal contractile force between circular and longitudinal muscle layers in the small intestine. However, the longitudinal muscle layer contracted more rapidly (75). With transection of the duodenum, variations in force ceased below the transection but showed periodic increases above. The number of spike potentials recorded simultaneously with force, and the duration of the spike bursts determined the magnitude of circular muscle contraction (10).

Nelsen and Becker were able to simulate intestinal electrical and mechanical events with a computer (71).

MOTOR ACTIVITY IN THE ILEUM

This portion of the small bowel is not readily accessible except in patients with ileostomies. Cummins studied five patients with small balloons introduced into the stoma. He found that evacuation of ileal contents was always associated with phasic contractions superimposed on a rise in tone. However, similar waves occurred in the absence of evacuation (27). Code et al. studied two patients and described a contraction of large amplitude, up to 80 to 100 cm H_2O (48), occurring simultaneously at separated points in the ileum (24). They were uncommon in the fasting state but increased markedly after a hearty breakfast (24).

THE ILEOCECAL VALVE

A high-pressure zone has been described at the ileocecal junction. In man the pressure measured 20 mm Hg on pull-through and was about 4 cm in length (25). When a balloon was inflated in the ileum in 41 of 47 trials, there was a mean drop of 70 per cent in the pressure in the sphincteric zone. Inflation in the colon caused a rise in pressure in 12 of 15 trials. In a patient with a transplanted segment including the sphincter, similar responses occurred (25). In animals sympathetic stimulation produced contraction while vagal stimulation gave equivocal results. The vagus may contain adrenergic fibers destined for beta receptors (55). Responses to distention similar to those described above have been reported in dogs (57).

ANALYSIS OF MOTILITY RECORDS

Various attempts have been made to simplify quantification of motility records (26,86). None have been generally satisfactory. Recently use of an off-line digitalizing computer has been reported to save time (68).

PRESSURE-FLOW RELATIONSHIPS

Injection of a bolus into a loop of intestine in an anesthetized dog resulted in a reduction of contractions and electrical spikes distal to the bolus but an increase cephalad. This response was abolished by 0.1 per cent cocaine in the lumen. A single injection of saline under 10 cm of water pressure resulted in a single outflow, but if HCl was injected outflow was retarded (69). In man, perfusion of an intestinal loop at a flow rate of 3 to 7 ml per minute resulted in distention of the segment to accommodate the flow. At levels above 7 ml per minute, the transit time shortened (31). Barriero et al. used a dye dilution technique to measure transit time in normal human subjects. They found a mean transit time of 12 minutes for a 25-cm segment (7). Propagated contraction waves shortened the transit time regardless of the wave form (8).

GRADIENTS OF INTESTINAL ACTIVITY

In general, the proximal small intestine shows greater activity than the distal whether the factor measured is slow-wave frequency, oxygen consumption, or mechanical contractions. Hasselbrack and Thomas confirmed the presence of duodenal influences increasing the frequency of rhythmic contractions below (43). No pacemaker analagous to the SA node in the heart has been identified. If a segment of duodenum is reversed, motility during the interdigestive phase and in response to cholinergic drugs and 5-hydroxytryptamine was reduced (65). However, transit of barium through the segment was not slowed. The gradient of contractile force may be responsible for transit. Hypoxia sufficient to destroy parts of the myenteric plexus but not the muscle was followed by failure of slow-wave activity to spread into the segment from adjacent normal areas. Slow waves within the segment spread in both cephalad and caudad directions (79). The frequency of mechanical contraction was reduced similarly (80).

Christensen and his associates recorded slow waves from the human small intestine. The frequency varied from 12 per minute in the duodenum to 9 in the ileum (22). The drop occurred in two steps rather than as a gradual fall—one at 90 to 120 cm and the second at 190 to 220 cm within the gastrointestinal tract (20). Patients with hyperthyroidism showed an increased frequency, those with hypothyroidism a decrease (21). Insulin hypoglycemia slowed the frequency. The authors concluded that slow waves reflected metabolic activity within the gut (23). Hyperthermia similarly increased frequency. In dogs, ligation of the intestine slowed the frequency of slow waves below the point of ligation by lengthening the duration of the slow waves (11). Despite years of effort the significance of the slow wave is obscure (12).

VILLIKININ

The intestinal villi exhibit a pumping action which may contribute to absorption. Intestinal extracts have been found to increase the contractile activity, and the task of purifying the material is under way (61). An inhibitor of villous motility can also be extracted from the mucosa (62).

LOCAL HORMONES AND INTESTINAL MOTILITY

A number of substances have been extracted from the intestine which have striking effects on intestinal motility. Their physiologic significance remains unknown. 5-Hydroxytryptamine or serotonin is one of these. It can be found in the mucosa and in the myenteric plexus. Almost complete depletion of mucosal serotonin fails to abolish the peristaltic reflex. After the administration of serotonin it can be identified in nerve endings (40). Intraarterial acetylcholine or increased intraluminal pressures released serotonin into the venous effluent of perfused segments of intestine (18). Human proximal jejunal segments in vitro contracted to low concentrations of serotonin (6). In man, serotonin increased motor activity in the small intestine (46). Other substances active on motor function are substance P, darmstoff, and prostaglandins (9).

ENDOCRINE INFLUENCES ON INTESTINAL MOTILITY

Glucagon inhibited jejunal motility in man whether given intravenously or intraportally (32,60). Cholecystokinin stimulated contractions in cat small intestine which was blocked by atropine (44). Bilateral adrenalectomy in rats accelerated small intestinal transit, possibly because of altered potassium balance (89). Kock found the release of epinephrine from the adrenal medulla to be an important factor in the inhibition of intestinal motility in the cat (59).

NERVOUS CONTROL OF INTESTINAL MOTILITY

Now that ganglion cells in the myenteric plexus have been approached with microelectrodes, some of the mysteries of the function of this structure may be dispelled (90). Action potentials from longitudinal muscle and the ganglion cells seemed to occur together. Tidball found that the tonus of isolated rabbit intestine was proportional to the amount of acetylcholine released into the bath (82). Epinephrine appeared to decrease the release of acetylcholine (81). Van Harn found that slow waves originated in longitudinal muscle. He showed that when the intestine was active, sympathetic stimulation caused hyperpolarization, cessation of spikes, and inhibition of contraction. When the intestine was inactive, stimulation of either the sympathetics or the vagus caused depolarization, initiation of spikes, and contraction. An increase in intraluminal pressure produced spikes and an increase in the amplitude and frequency of contractions. He suggested that in the quiescent muscle adrenergic receptors were occupied already. Both excitatory and inhibitory fibers may be present in both divisions of the autonomic nervous system (83).

In dogs, denervation of the duodenum by complete excision and autologous reinsertion had no effect on contractile activity (28). There was no significant difference in the motor behavior of innervated and denervated Thiry-Vella loops in dogs (47). In man bilateral vagotomy produced an increase in the frequency of bursts of phasic contractions superimposed upon a rise of baseline (76).

Distention of an area of the intestine produces inhibition of contractile activity elsewhere in the intestine—the intestinointestinal inhibitory reflex (91). Hukuhara et al. distinguished between a mucosal reflex which produced inhibition caudad and excited proximally, and a muscular stimulation which inhibited on both sides (51). The receptor for the latter was thought to be located in the longitudinal muscle layer. Its cell body may lie in the myenteric plexus where it may synapse with the inhibitory neuron. The mucosal reflex involved a spinal neuron (52). There is considerable debate over whether the inhibitory reflex must involve spinal pathways or whether it might act through a prevertebral sympathetic ganglion (91).

Vagal stimulation can result in either excitation or inhibition of motility. Weak stimulation caused excitation only. Atropine converted excitation to inhibition. There may be two kinds of effector neurons in the myenteric plexus, both in synaptic connection with the vagus (70). In cats, Kewenter found that vagal stimulation excited the jejunum but had little effect on the ileum. He noted that there were inhibitory fibers to the ileum in the splanchnics and no vagal inhibitory fibers at the level of the neck. The inhibitory fibers were high threshold and caused a decrease in blood flow on stimulation. Therefore the stimulus strength determined the character of the response (58). Johansson et al. found that supraspinal structures exerted an inhibitory influence on spinal transmission of the intestinointestinal inhibitory reflex (56).

McCoy and Baker found that feeding stabilized electrical activity of the small intestine (67). Sham feeding increased the motility of a duodenal pouch (72). Physical training increased propulsive activity in rats, and sleep was associated with a clear decrease of small intestinal motility in 12 of 16 subjects (45,85).

PHARMACOLOGY OF INTESTINAL MOTILITY

The concept of alpha and beta receptors arose from the observation that the actions of norepinephrine and isoprenaline could be selectively blocked. In the intestine, the canine ileum responds to both agents with relaxation which is subject to blockade by the appropriate antagonists (1). Bennett and Whitney made the general observation that the intrinsic nerves were relatively inactive in the stomach and proximal duodenum. Cholinergic drive was dominant in the distal duodenum and jejunum, while in the ileum and colon the dominant influence was sympathetic (15). Isolated human jejunal longitudinal muscle strips contracted in response to acetylcholine and relaxed in response to norepinephrine and isoprenaline (88). Electrical recordings may be helpful in the interpretation of drug actions (87).

CIRCULATORY EFFECTS

Ligation of the superior mesenteric artery in dogs led to increased intra-luminal pressures in the jejunum in six of seven animals. With superior mesenteric venous ligation there was a marked increase in amplitude of pressure waves (92).

PATHOPHYSIOLOGY

Motor disorders of the small intestine may result in diarrhea or constipation. In general, anticholinergic drugs slow intestinal transit, while cholinergic agents stimulate propulsive activity.

Motility of the Gallbladder and Biliary Tree

The mechanism by which bile passes from the thin-walled gallbladder into the common bile duct and past the resistance of the sphincter of Oddi and the duodenal wall is a fascinating example of coordinated control. For many years it was considered to be the result of "reciprocal innervation," with contraction of the gallbladder coordinated with relaxation of the sphincter of Oddi via a nervous reflex mechanism. More recently the observation that the hormone cholecystokinin produced both of these effects seemed to remove the necessity for nervous control (67b).

Purification of the hormone by Jorpes and Mutt (56a) led to the identification of a polypeptide containing 33 amino acids. The sequence of the C-terminal octapeptide has been determined. Interestingly, the C-terminal tetrapeptide is identical with that of gastrin. An even less likely parallel exists with a decapeptide isolated from the skin of an Australian frog. This substance, caerulein, differs from cholecystokinin by only one amino acid. In terms of its potency in causing contraction of the gallbladder, caerulein is 8 to 16 times as potent as cholecystokinin, while gastrin is only one thirtieth as potent (82a). This suggests that endogenous gastrin has little physiologic significance in the control of gallbladder emptying. These studies have confirmed the identity of cholecystokinin and pancreozymin.

Recent studies suggest that a neuronal control of evacuation of the gallbladder exists. Snape showed some years ago that, in conscious dogs, vagotomy led to a doubling of the latent period for emptying of the gallbladder after intraduodenal food products (78b). There was no change in the responsiveness of the gallbladder to cholecystokinin (78a). Complete vagotomy in dogs and man led to a significant increase in the area of the gallbladder silhouette as seen radiographically after contrast media (76a,76b).

In anesthetized dogs, Wyatt found that mechanical or electrical stimulation of the gallbladder led to contraction of the gallbladder and relaxation of the sphincter of Oddi. This effect did not occur following excision of the celiac ganglion or infiltration of the periductal tissues with procaine (87a,87b).

Isolated human gallbladder muscle exhibited spontaneous contractions in vitro. Acetylcholine caused a sustained contraction which was abolished by atropine. Cholecystokinin produced contraction of a similar amplitude but after a longer latent period. Atropine did not affect the contraction (67a).

Changes in the capacity and emptying of the gallbladder occur during the menstrual cycle and pregnancy. Oral cholecystograms done on the fourteenth and twenty-first days of the menstrual cycle showed a reduction in emptying in response to cholecystokinin on the twenty-first day which was attributed to the action of progesterone (71a).

PATHOPHYSIOLOGY

The gallbladder, by virtue of its role as a reservoir, acts to decompress the biliary tree. In dogs, after ligation of the common bile duct, the serum bilirubin rises much more slowly if the gallbladder is present. There is a prompt gush of bile under considerable pressure from the common bile duct after catheterization of the sphincter of Oddi in dogs, if the gallbladder has been removed. If the gallbladder is present, bile may not appear for up to an hour.

There has been much speculation over the possibility that failure of relaxation of the sphincter to occur concomitantly with contraction of the gallbladder could lead to pain simulating partial obstruction of the common bile duct—"biliary dyskinesia." While the existence of the snydrome is debated, present evidence does not exclude the possibility.

Stasis in other hollow organs favors the formation of calculi. It may be that the hormonal changes in pregnancy leading to delayed gallbladder emptying contribute to the formation of gallstones.

References

1. Ahlquist, R. P., and B. Levy. Adrenergic receptive mechanism of canine ileum. *J. Pharmacol. Exp. Ther.* **127:** 146–149, 1959.
2. Allen, G. L., E. W. Poole, and C. F. Code. Relationships between electrical activities of antrum and duodenum. *Am. J. Physiol.* **207:** 906–910, 1964.
3. Andersson, S., and M. I. Grossman. Profile of pH, pressure and potential difference at gastroduodenal junction in man. *Gastroenterology* **49:** 364–371, 1965.
4. Atkinson, M., D. A. W. Edwards, A. J. Honour, and E. N. Rowlands. Comparison of cardiac and pyloric sphincters. *Lancet* **2:** 918–922, 1957.
5. Barany, F., and B. Jacobson. Endoradiosonde study of propulsion and pressure activity induced by test meals, prostigmine, and diphenoxylate in the small intestine. *Gut* **5:** 90–95, 1964.
6. Barbero, G. J., I. C. Kim, and J. Davis. Duodenal motility patterns in infants and children. *Pediatrics* **22:** 1054–1063, 1958.
7. Barriero, M. A., R. D. McKenna, and I. T. Beck. Determination of transit time in the human jejunum by the single-injection of indicator dilution technic. *Am. J. Dig. Dis.* **13:** 222–233, 1968.
8. Barriero, M. A., R. D. McKenna, and I. T. Beck. The physiologic significance of intraluminal pressure changes in relation to propulsion and absorption in the human jejunum. *Am. J. Dig. Dis.* **13:** 234–251, 1968.
9. Bass, P., and D. R. Bennett. Local chemical regulation of motor action of the bowel; substance P and lipid-soluble acids. In: *Handbook of Physiology.* Section 6: Alimentary Tract. Vol. IV: Motility. Edited by C. F. Code. Washington, D.C.: American Physiological Society, 1968, pp. 2193–2212.
10. Bass, P., and J. N. Wiley. Electrical and extraluminal contractile-force activity in duodenum of the dog. *Am. J. Dig. Dis.* **10:** 183–200, 1965.
11. Bass, P., and J. N. Wiley. Effects of ligation and morphine on electric and motor activity of dog duodenum. *Am. J. Physiol.* **208:** 908–913, 1965.
12. Bass, P. In vivo electrical activity of the small bowel. In: *Handbook of Physiology.* Section 6: Alimentary Tract. Vol. IV: Motility. Edited by C. F. Code. Washington, D.C.: American Physiological Society, 1968, pp. 2051–2074.
13. Beck, I. T., R. D. McKenna, G. Peterfy, J. Sidorov, and H. Strawczrnski. Pressure studies in the normal human jejunum. *Am. J. Dig. Dis.* **10:** 436–448, 1965.
14. Beleslin, D. B., S. B. Bogdanovic, and M. M. Rakic. The effect of morphine and anticholinesterases on the peristaltic reflex of the isolated guinea pig ileum. *Arch. Int. Pharmacodyn.* **149:** 457–466, 1964.

15. Bennett, A., and B. Whitney. A pharmacological study of the motility of the human gastrointestinal tract. *Gut* **7**: 307–316, 1966.

16. Bessou, P., and E. R. Perl. A movement receptor of the small intestine. *J. Physiol.* **182**: 404–426, 1966.

17. Brink, B. M., J. F. Schlegel, and C. F. Code. The pressure profile of the gastroduodenal junctional zone in dogs. *Gut* **6**: 163–171, 1965.

18. Burks, T. F., and J. P. Long. 5-Hydroxytryptamine release into dog intestinal vasculature. *Am. J. Physiol.* **211**: 619–625, 1966.

19. Carlson, H. C., C. F. Code, and R. A. Nelson. Motor action of the canine gastroduodenal junction: A cineradiographic, pressure and electric study. *Am. J. Dig. Dis.* **11**: 155–172, 1966.

20. Christenson, J., H. P. Schedl, and J. A. Clifton. The small intestinal basic electrical rhythm in man: (BER) Its frequency and gradient. *Gastroenterology* **46**: 773–774, 1964.

21. Christenson, J., H. P. Schedl, and J. A. Clifton. The basic electrical rhythm of the duodenum in normal human subjects and in patients with thyroid disease. *J. Clin. Invest.* **43**: 1659–1667, 1964.

22. Christensen, J., H. P. Schedl., and J. A. Clifton. The small intestinal basic electrical rhythm (slow wave), frequency gradient in normal men and in patients with a variety of diseases. *Gastroenterology* **50**: 309–315, 1966.

23. Christensen, J., J. A. Clifton, and H. P. Schedl. Variations in the frequency of the human duodenal basic electrical rhythm in health and disease. *Gastroenterology* **51**: 200–206, 1966.

24. Code, C. F., A. G. Rogers, J. Schlegel, N. C. Hightower, Jr., and J. A. Bargen. Motility patterns in the terminal ileum: Studies on two patients with ulcerative colitis and ileac stomas. *Gastroenterology* **32**: 651–665, 1957.

25. Cohen, S., L. D. Harris, and R. Levitan. Manometric characteristics of the human ileocecal junctional zone. *Gastroenterology* **54**: 72–75, 1968.

26. Connell, A. M., E. C. Texter, Jr., and G. Vantrappen. Classification and interpretation of motility records. *Am. J. Dig. Dis.* **10**: 481–483, 1965.

27. Cummins, A. J. Small intestinal function in patients with an ileostomy. *Am. J. Med.* **16**: 237–245, 1954.

28. Dancer, J. T., W. D. Hawley, and M. K. DuVal. The intrinsic contractile activity of the duodenum. *Arch. Surg.* **88**: 984–987, 1964.

29. Daniel, E. E., and G. E. Wieba. Transmission of reflexes arising on both sides of the gastroduodenal junction. *Am. J. Physiol.* **211**: 634–642, 1966.

30. Deller, D. J., and A. G. Wangel. Intestinal motility in man. I. A study combining the use of intraluminal pressure recording and cineradiography. *Gastroenterology* **48**: 45–57, 1965.

31. Dillard, R. L., H. Eastman, and J. S. Fordtran. Volume-flow relationship during the transport of fluid through the human small intestine. *Gastroenterology* **49**: 58–66, 1965.

32. Dotevall, G., and N. G. Kock. The effect of glucagon on intestinal motility in man. *Gastroenterology* **45**: 364–367, 1963.

33. Edwards, D. A. W., and E. N. Rowlands. Physiology of the gastroduodenal junction. In: *Handbook of Physiology*. Section 6: Alimentary Tract. Vol. IV: Motility. Edited by C. F. Code. Washington, D.C.: American Physiological Society, 1968, pp. 1985–2000.

34. Farrar, J. T., and A. M. Zfass. Small intestinal motility. *Gastroenterology* **52:** 1019–1037, 1967.
35. Fink, S. The intraluminal pressures in the intact human intestine. *Gastroenterology* **36:** 661–671, 1959.
36. Fishlock, D. J., A. G. Parks, and J. V. Dewell. Action of 5-hydroxytryptamine on the human stomach, duodenum and jejunum in vitro. *Gut* **6:** 338–342, 1965.
37. Foulk, W. T., C. F. Code, C. G. Morlock, and J. A. Bargen. A study of the motility patterns and the basic rhythm in the duodenum and upper part of the jejunum of human beings. *Gastroenterology* **26:** 601–611, 1954.
38. Friedman, G., J. D. Waye, L. A. Weingarten, and H. D. Janowitz. The pattern of simultaneous intraluminal pressure changes in the human proximal small intestine. *Gastroenterology* **47:** 258–268, 1964.
39. Friedman, G., B. S. Wolf, J. D. Waye, and H. D. Janowitz. Correlation of cineradiographic and intraluminal pressure changes in the human duodenum: an analysis of the functional significance of monophasic waves. *Gastroenterology* **49:** 37–49, 1965.
40. Gershon, M. D. Serotonin and the motility of the gastrointestinal tract. *Gastroenterology* **54:** 453–456, 1968.
41. Ghormley, R. K., N. C. Hightower, Jr., C. F. Code, and J. T. Priestley. Observations on intestinal motility through a paper-thin abdominal wall 14 years after removal of epithelioma; report of a case. *Mayo Clin. Proc.* **29:** 311–316, 1954.
42. Hansky, J., and A. M. Connell. Measurement of gastrointestinal transit using radioactive chromium. *Gut* **3:** 187–188, 1962.
43. Hasselbrack, R., and J. E. Thomas. Control of intestinal rhythmic contractions by a duodenal pacemaker. *Am. J. Physiol.* **201:** 955–960, 1961.
44. Hedner, P., H. Persson, and G. Rorsman. Effect of cholecystokinin on small intestine. *Acta Physiol. Scand.* **70:** 250–254, 1967.
45. Helm, J. D., Jr., P. Kramer, R. M. MacDonald, and F. J. Inglefinger. Changes in motility of the human small intestine during sleep. *Gastroenterology* **10:** 135–137, 1948.
46. Hendrix, T. R., M. Atkinson, J. A. Clifton, and F. J. Inglefinger. The effect of 5-hydroxytryptamine on intestinal motor function in man. *Am. J. Med.* **23:** 886–893, 1957.
47. Hiatt, R. B., I. Goodman, and R. Bircher. Control of motility in Thiry-Vella ileal segments in dogs. *Am. J. Physiol.* **210:** 373–378, 1966.
48. Hightower, N. C., Jr. Motility of the alimentary canal of man. In: *Disturbances in Gastrointestinal Motility.* Edited by J. A. Rider and H. C. Moeller. Springfield, Ill.: Charles C Thomas, 1959, pp. 3–61.
49. Hightower, N. C., Jr. Motor action of the small bowel. In: *Handbook of Physiology.* Section 6: Alimentary Tract. Vol. IV: Motility. Edited by C. F. Code. Washington, D.C.: American Physiological Society, 1968, pp. 2001–2024.
50. Horowitz, L., and J. T. Farrar. Intraluminal small intestinal pressures in normal patients and in patients with functional gastrointestinal disorders. *Gastroenterology* **42:** 455–464, 1962.
51. Hukuhara, T., M. Yamagami, and S. Nakayama. On the intestinal intrinsic reflexes. *Jap. J. Physiol.* **8:** 9–20, 1958.
52. Hukuhara, T., S. Nakayama, and R. Namba. Locality of receptors concerned with the intestino-intestinal extrinsic and intestinal muscular intrinsic reflexes. *Jap. J. Physiol.* **10:** 414–419, 1960.

53. Hukuhara, T., and H. Fukuda. The motility of the isolated guinea-pig small intestine. *Jap. J. Physiol.* **15:** 125–139, 1965.

54. Jacoby, H. I., P. Bass, and D. R. Bennett. In vivo extraluminal contractile force transducer for gastrointestinal muscle. *J. Appl. Physiol.* **18:** 658–665, 1963.

55. Jarrett, R. J., and J. C. Gazet. Studies in vivo of the ileocaeco-colic sphincter in the cat and dog. *Gut* **7:** 271–276, 1966.

56. Johansson, B., O. Jonsson, and B. Ljung. Supraspinal control of the intestino-intestinal inhibitory reflex. *Acta Physiol. Scand.* **63:** 442–449, 1965.

56a. Jorpes, J. E. The isolation and chemistry of secretin and cholecystokinin. *Gastroenterology* **55:** 157–164, 1968.

57. Kelley, M. L., Jr., E. A. Gordon, and J. A. Deweese. Pressure responses of canine ileocolonic junctional zone to intestinal distention. *Am. J. Physiol.* **211:** 614–618, 1966.

58. Kewenter, J. The vagal control of the jejunal and ileal motility and blood flow. *Acta Physiol Scand.* Suppl. **251:** 1–68, 1965.

59. Kock, N. G. An experimental analysis of mechanisms engaged in reflex inhibition of intestinal motility. *Acta Physiol. Scand.* Suppl. **164:** 1–54, 1959.

60. Kock, N. G., N. Darle, and G. Dotevall. Inhibition of intestinal motility in man by glucagon given intraportally. *Gastroenterology* **53:** 88–92, 1967.

61. Kokas, E., and C. L. Johnston, Jr. Influence of refined villikinin on motility of intestinal villi. *Am. J. Physiol.* **208:** 1196–1202, 1965.

62. Kokas, E., and C. L. Johnston Jr. Evidence for an intestinal inhibitor of villous motility. *Arch. Int. Pharmacodyn.* **160:** 211–222, 1966.

63. Kosterlitz, H. W. Intrinsic and extrinsic nervous control of motility of the stomach and the intestine. In: *Handbook of Physiology.* Section 6: Alimentary Tract. Vol. IV: Motility. Edited by C. F. Code. Washington, D.C.: American Physiological Society, 1968, pp. 2147–2171.

64. Lish, P. M., B. B. Clark, and S. I. Robbins. Effects of some physiologic substances on gastrointestinal propulsion in the rat. *Am. J. Physiol.* **197:** 22–26, 1959.

65. Ludwick, J. R., J. N. Wiley, and P. Bass. Extraluminal contractile force and electrical activity of reversed canine duodenum. *Gastroenterology* **54:** 41–51, 1968.

66. McCance, R. A., K. M. Prior, and E. W. Widdowson. A radiological study of the rate of passage of brown and white bread through the digestive tract of man. *Brit. J. Nutr.* **7:** 98–104, 1953.

67. McCoy, E. J., and R. D. Baker. Effect of feeding on electrical activity of dog's small intestine. *Am. J. Physiol.* **214:** 1291–1295, 1968.

67a. Mack, A. J., and J. K. Todd. A study of human gall bladder muscle in vitro. *Gut* **9:** 546–549, 1968.

67b. Magee, D. F. Physiology of gallbladder emptying. In *The Biliary System,* edited by W. Taylor. Oxford: Blackwell Scientific Publications, 1965, pp. 233–247.

68. Misiewicz, J. J., S. L. Waller, M. J. R. Healy, and E. A. Piper. Computer analysis of intraluminal pressure records. *Gut* **9:** 232–236, 1968.

69. Nakayama, S. Movements of small intestine in transport of intraluminal contents. *Jap. J. Physiol.* **12:** 522–533, 1962.

70. Nakayama, S. The effects of stimulation of the vagus nerve on movements of the small intestine. *Jap. J. Physiol.* **15:** 243–252, 1965.

71. Nelsen, T. S., and J. C. Becker. Simulation of the electrical and mechanical gradient of the small intestine. *Am. J. Physiol.* **214:** 749–757, 1968.

71a. Nilsson, S., and S. Stattin. Gallbladder emptying during the normal menstrual cycle. *Acta Chir. Scand.* **133**: 648–652, 1967.

72. Preshaw, R. M., and R. S. Knauf. The effect of sham feeding on the secretion and motility of canine duodenal pouches. *Gastroenterology* **51**: 193–199, 1966.

73. Ramorino, M. L., and C. Colagrande. Intestinal motility. Preliminary studies with telemetering capsules and synchronized fluorocinematography. *Am. J. Dig. Dis.* **9**: 64–71, 1964.

74. Reinke, D. A., A. H. Rosenbaum, and D. R. Bennett. Patterns of dog gastrointestinal contractile activity monitored in vivo with extraluminal force transducers. *Am. J. Dig. Dis.* **12**: 113–141, 1967.

75. Rosenbaum, A. H., D. A. Reinke, and D. R. Bennett. In vivo force, frequency and velocity of dog gastrointestinal contractile activity. *Am. J. Dig. Dis.* **12**: 142–153, 1967.

76. Roth, H. P., and A. J. Beams. The effect of vagotomy on the motility of the small intestine. *Gastroenterology* **36**: 452–458, 1959.

76a. Rudick, J., and J. S. F. Hutchison. Effects of vagal-nerve section on the biliary system. *Lancet* **1**: 579–581, 1964.

76b. Scheinin, T. M., M. V. Inberg, and E. Lehtinen. Effect of selective gastric and total abdominal vagotomy on the canine gallbladder. *Ann. Med. Exp. Biol. Fenn.* **45**: 377–380, 1967.

77. Schofield, G. C. Anatomy of muscular and neural tissues in the alimentary canal. In: *Handbook of Physiology.* Section 6, Vol. IV: Motility. Edited C. F. Code. Washington, D.C.: American Physiological Society, 1968, pp. 1579–1627.

78. Smith, H. W., and E. C. Texter, Jr. Characteristics of the phasic intraluminal pressure waves of the stomach and duodenum. *Am. J. Dig. Dis.* **12**: 318–326, 1957.

78a. Snape, W. J., M. H. F. Friedman, and J. E. Thomas. The assay of cholecystokinin and the influence of vagotomy on the gallbladder, *Gastroenterology* **10**: 496–501, 1948.

78b. Snape, W. J. Studies on the gall-bladder in unanesthetized dogs before and after vagotomy. *Gastroenterology* **10**: 129–134, 1948.

79. Szurszewski, J., and F. R. Steggerda. The effect of hypoxia on the electrical slow wave of the canine small intestine. *Am. J. Dig. Dis.* **13**: 168–177, 1968.

80. Szurszewski, J., and F. R. Steggerda. The effect of hypoxia on the mechanical activity of the canine small intestine. *Am. J. Dig. Dis.* **13**: 178–185, 1968.

81. Tidball, M. E. Effect of epinephrine on relation of acetylcholine to intestinal tonus. *Am. J. Physiol.* **197**: 1327–1329, 1959.

82. Tidball, M. E. Relationship between acetylcholine and tonus in isolated rabbit intestine. *Am. J. Physiol.* **197**: 561–564, 1959.

82. Vagne, M., and M. I. Grossman. Effect of gastrin on motility of gallbladder. *Physiologist* **10**: 330, 1967.

83. Van Harn, G. L. Responses of muscles of cat small intestine to autonomic nerve stimulation. *Am. J. Physiol.* **204**: 352–358, 1963.

84. Van Liere, E. J., H. H. Hess, and J. E. Edwards. Effect of physical training on propulsive motility of the small intestine. *J. Appl. Physiol.* **7**: 186–187, 1954.

85. Vantrappen, G., J. Hellemans, and J. Vandenbroucke. A method for the analysis of intestinal motility records. *Am. J. Dig. Dis.* **10**: 449–454, 1965.

86. Vaughan Williams, E. M. The mode of action of drugs upon intestinal motility. *Pharmacol. Rev.* **6**: 159–190, 1954.

87. Whitney, B. A preliminary investigation of the pharmacology of longitudinal muscle strips from human isolated jejunum. *J. Pharm. Pharmacol.* **17**: 465–473, 1965.

87a. Wyatt, A. P., F. O. Belzer, and J. E. Dunphy. Malfunction without constriction of the common bile duct. *Am. J. Surg.* **113**: 592–598, 1967.

87b. Wyatt, A. P. The relationship of the sphincter of Oddi to the stomach, duodenum and gallbladder. *J. Physiol. London* **193**: 225–243, 1967.

88. Wyman, L. C. The effect of adrenalectomy on propulsive motility of the small intestine in rats. *Proc. Soc. Exp. Biol. Med.* **84**: 303–304, 1953.

89. Yokoyama, S. Aktions potentiale der Ganglienzelle des Auerbachschen Plexus in Kaninchendunndarm. *Pflügers Arch. Ges. Physiol.* **288**: 95–102, 1966.

90. Youmans, W. B. Innervation of the gastrointestinal tract. In: *Handbook of Physiology.* Section 6: Alimentary Tract. Vol. IV: Motility. Edited by C. F. Code. Washington, D.C.: American Physiological Society, 1968, pp. 1655–1663.

91. Zfass, A. M., L. Horowitz, and J. T. Farrar. Effect of vascular occlusion on small-bowel intraluminal pressures in dogs. *Am. J. Dig. Dis.* **12**: 154–161, 1967.

CHAPTER

Colonic Motility

THE COLON is primarily a collection point for the intestinal stream which periodically transports the contents from the right side to the left side of the colon. Between these mass movements the colonic contents are kneaded and shifted to and fro between haustra which probably facilitates the absorption of water. In contrast to the small intestine, there is little propulsive activity except for the mass movements which have been estimated to occur no more frequently than once or twice a day.

Structural Basis for Colonic Motility

The characteristic feature of the colon is the presence of sacculations or haustra connected by muscular bands or taenia. While some haustral folds disappear when the taenia are cut, others persist until the serosa has been incised (51). The problems of innervation are similar to those elsewhere in the gut. In the mouse colon, there were no intimate relationships between nerve endings and either epithelial or muscle cells (48).

Human Colon In Vitro

Circular and longitudinal muscle from human colon contracted in response to nicotine, suggesting that both adrenergic and cholinergic systems were

192

present (53). Bucknell and Clark describe a human preparation for the study of the peristaltic reflex in vitro (7).

Colonic Motility

The problems of the interpretation of records of colonic motility are similar to those elsewhere (8). Connell does not express much enthusiasm for computer methodology (17). In the sigmoid colon, contractile waves, when rhythmic, occur at the rate of two per minute and with an amplitude of 5 to 100 cm H_2O. Characteristically there are periods of activity and inactivity lasting about 30 minutes. Records as little as 1 cm apart are dissimilar. Conducted waves are rare and do not necessarily indicate propulsion. The major function of such contractions is probably to retard flow (15). Using miniature balloons in the pelvic colon, Connell found that activity was present 50 per cent of the time. Compared to the sigmoid, the amplitude of waves in the rectum was less. Day-to-day variations in the same patient may reach 90 per cent (11). Using open-tipped catheters, Chaudhary and Truelove found activity present 13 per cent of the time in the sigmoid (9). There are difficulties in keeping catheters patent even with slow perfusions. Fink recorded from the cecum in two patients and found phasic waves present 40 to 50 per cent of the time, while in the sigmoid activity varied from 15 to 90 per cent of time (21). Kock et al. recorded from both right colon and sigmoid and found that after feeding and prostigmine the activity of the sigmoid was greater than that on the right side of the colon (34).

In two studies in children with catheters, the pressure waves were of lower amplitude in the rectum than in the sigmoid (19). Activity was present 47 per cent of the time, and less in infants under six months of age. Activity was less with repeated studies, and anxious subjects showed more activity (10).

Combined pressure sensing and cineradiography confirmed an increase in motor activity with eating and prostigmine (20,38). Gaseous contents in the colon moved more rapidly than propulsive contractions. Liquid contents seemed to leak through after a contraction when the walls were at a low tone. Most propulsive activity carried so much gas ahead that tandem tips registered pressure changes simultaneously. Solid or semisolid content was transported only when resistance was low. The observers saw only one peristaltic wave in 200 studies.

Telemetering devices have the advantage of passing readily into the colon. They were usually passed within 48 hours. A comparison of activity on the right and left side of the colon showed higher amplitude and longer duration waves on the right but greater overall activity on the left (5). Ramorino and Colagrande saw no phasic contractions superimposed on an increase in baseline above the sigmoid (44). Eating increased activity in the colon from 18 to 29 per cent of the time. Force transducers also confirmed the stimulating effect of eating in dogs (45).

Evacuation of the Colon

After barium by mouth, the meal reaches the rectum and colon in about 24 hours. There was a tendency for barium to accumulate in the left colon (35). There is no better description of mass movements than the original by Holzknecht. He saw disappearance of haustrations and sudden movement of the barium column from the right to left colon. Then the segmentation reappeared. The subject was unaware of the events. He saw such movements twice in 1,000 studies (28).

Humoral Effects on Colonic Motility

Serotonin inhibited motor activity in the human colon in vivo (39). Similar effects were noted in vitro (37). Serotonin probably acts directly on colonic muscle. Bradykinin had a similar effect (40).

Nervous Control of Colonic Motility

Japanese workers have transplanted free autographs of the colon to the esophagus. Following a brief period of vigorous peristalsis, activity gradually fell to a very low level. Histologic studies showed degeneration of the cells of the myenteric plexus (41). This suggests that normal innervation is necessary for the usual degree of activity. In the cat there was no pharmacologic evidence for parasympathetic ganglion cells in the wall of the colon. Autonomic control seemed to be mediated through the sympathetics. Sympathetic inhibition was mediated mainly through beta receptors.

Gillespie found that single stimuli to the sympathetic nerves were ineffective on the rabbit colon. Repetitive stimulation was followed by complete electrical and mechanical quiescence. Inhibition may be due to stabilization of the membrane potential (24). Stimulation of pelvic nerves increased the amplitude of contraction while that of lumbar nerves led to inhibition (23). Single stimuli to pelvic nerves caused depolarization to single cells (25). All cells studied responded to stimulation of either right or left pelvic nerve (26,27).

In anesthetized dogs, stroking the mucosa after cutting inhibitory nerves led to relaxation below and contraction above the point of stimulation. Muscles responded by inhibition on both sides, as described earlier in the small intestine (29).

In man, Fink found that methacholine increased phasic activity on the right side of the colon and suggested that there might be more cholinesterase on the left side (22). In another study, acetylcholine intravenously caused contraction of the right colon and inhibition of activity on the left (33).

In patients with complete destruction of the lumbosacral spinal cord there was greater pressure activity than in normals or in patients with higher transections. Low cord destruction abolished all reflex activity including the intestinointestinal inhibitory reflex (13). Stimulation of the forebrain in the cat gave variable effects on colonic motility (31). Section of the spinal cord at L-6 abolished most effects of brain stimulation. Implantation of crystals of acetylcholine in the anterior hypothalamus led to inhibition of colonic activity most of the time (6). In a series of papers using the stressful interview technique, Almy and his colleagues produced changes in colonic motility. Patients with weeping and feelings of hopelessness usually showed decreased activity in the sigmoid (4). Pain, on the other hand, usually elicited an increase in activity (2,3). Proctoscopy in medical students during a stressful interview showed increased contraction (1). Sleep and amobarbital reduced sigmoid motility (47). The relationship between pressure and volume for the sigmoid can be determined (36).

The most important conclusion from these studies is that colonic contents flow in response to a pressure gradient and that the effect of much of the segmenting activity is to retard rather than accelerate passage of content (18,52).

Pathophysiology

Diarrhea may be expected to be associated with reduced phasic activity in the left side of the colon (12,32,50). Some patients with abdominal pain after meals fail to show any change in mean activity in the sigmoid after eating. In diverticulitis, the pressure within the involved segments may be abnormally high. Drugs such as morphine may increase it still further (43). A lesion resembling congenital megacolon can be produced by perfusing a segment of colon with Tyrode's solution for several hours with the resultant hypoxic destruction of ganglion cells (30). Connell concludes that the main contribution of studies of colonic motility to clinical medicine has been in the area of concepts rather than diagnostic procedures (16).

References

1. Almy, T. P., and M. Tulin. Alterations in colonic function in man under stress: Experimental production of changes simulating the irritable colon. *Gastroenterology* 8: 616–626, 1947.

2. Almy, T. P., F. Kern, Jr., and M. Tulin. Alteration in colonic function in man under stress. II. Experimental production of sigmoid spasm in healthy persons. *Gastroenterology* **12:** 425–436, 1949.

3. Almy, T. P., L. E. Hinkle, Jr., B. Berle, and F. Kern, Jr. Alterations in colonic function in man under stress. III. Experimental production of sigmoid spasm in patients with spastic constipation. *Gastroenterology* **12:** 437–449, 1949.

4. Almy, T. P., F. K. Abbot, and L. E. Hinkle, Jr. Alterations in colonic function in man under stress. IV. Hypomotility of the sigmoid colon and its relationship to the mechanism of functional diarrhea. *Gastroenterology* **15:** 95–103, 1950.

5. Bloom, A. A., P. LoPresti, and J. T. Farrar. Motility of the intact human colon. *Gastroenterology* **54:** 232–240, 1968.

6. Boom, R., G. Chavez-Ibarra, J. J. Del Villar, and R. Hernandez-Peón. Changes of colonic motility induced by electrical and chemical stimulation of the forebrain and hypothalamus in cats. *Int. J. Neuropharmacol.* **4:** 169–175, 1965.

7. Bucknell, A., and C. Clark. An experimental method for recording the behavior of human isolated colonic segments. *Gut* **8:** 569–573, 1967.

8. Chaudhary, N. A., and S. C. Truelove. Colonic motility: A critical review of methods and results. *Am. J. Med.* **31:** 86–106, 1961.

9. Chaudhary, N. A., and S. C. Truelove. Human colonic motility: A comparative study of normal subjects, patients with ulcerative colitis and patients with the irritable colon syndrome. *Gastroenterology* **40:** 1–17, 1961.

10. Chin-Kim, I., and G. J. Barbero. The pattern of rectosigmoid motility in children. *Gastroenterology* **45:** 57–66, 1963.

11. Connell, A. M. The motility of the pelvic colon. I. Motility in normals and patients with asymptomatic duodenal ulcer. *Gut* **2:** 175–186, 1961.

12. Connell, A. M. The motility of the pelvic colon. Part II. Paradoxical motility in diarrhoea and constipation. *Gut* **3:** 342–348, 1962.

13. Connell, A. M., H. Frankel, and L. Guttman. The motility of the pelvic colon following complete lesions of the spinal cord. *Paraplegia* **1:** 98–115, 1963.

14. Connell, A. M., F. Avery Jones, and E. N. Rowlands. Motility of the pelvic colon. Part IV. Abdominal pain associated with colonic hypermotility after meals. *Gut* **6:** 105–112, 1965.

15. Connell, A. M. Significance of pressure waves of the sigmoid colon. *Am. J. Dig. Dis.* **10:** 455–462, 1965.

16. Connell, A. M. Recording of intestinal motility: Routine or research? *Gut* **8:** 527–529, 1967.

17. Connell, A. M. Problems of methodology and interpretation and analysis of records. *Am. J. Dig. Dis.* **13:** 397–405, 1968.

18. Connell, A. M. Motor action of the large bowel. In: *Handbook of Physiology.* Section 6: Alimentary Tract. Vol. IV: Motility. Edited by C. F. Code. Washington, D.C.: American Physiological Society, 1968, pp. 2075–2091.

19. Davidson, M., M. H. Sleisenger, T. P. Almy, and S. Z. Levine. Studies of distal colonic motility in Children. I. Non-propulsive patterns in normal children. *Pediatrics* **17:** 807–819, 1956.

20. Deller, D. J., and A. G. Wangel. Intestinal motility in man. I. A study combining the use of intraluminal pressure recording and cineradiography. *Gastroenterology* **48:** 45–57, 1965.

21. Fink, S. The intraluminal pressures in the intact human intestine. *Gastroenterology* **36:** 661–671, 1959.

22. Fink, S., and G. Friedman. The differential effect of drugs on the proximal and distal colon. *Am. J. Med.* **28**: 534–540, 1960.
23. Gillespie, J. S., and B. R. Mackenna. The inhibitory action of the sympathetic nerves on the smooth muscle of the rabbit gut, its reversal by reserpine and restoration by catecholamines and by dopa. *J. Physiol. London* **156**: 17–34, 1961.
24. Gillespie, J. S. Spontaneous, mechanical and electrical activity of stretched and unstretched intestinal smooth muscle cells and their response to sympathetic nerve stimulation. *J. Physiol.* **162**: 54–75, 1962.
25. Gillespie, J. S. The electrical and mechanical responses of intestinal smooth muscle cells to stimulation of their extrinsic parasympathetic nerves. *J. Physiol.* **162**: 76–92, 1962.
26. Gillespie, J. S., and A. J. Mack. The electrical response of intestinal smooth muscle to stimulation of the extrinsic or intrinsic motor nerves. *J. Physiol.* **170**: 19–20P, 1964.
27. Gillespie, J. S. Electrical activity in the colon. In: *Handbook of Physiology.* Section 6: Alimentary Tract. Vol. IV: Motility. Edited by C. F. Code. Washington, D.C.: American Physiological Society, 1968, pp. 2093–2120.
28. Holzknecht, G. Die normale peristaltik des kolon. *Munchen. Med. Wschr.* **56**: 2401–2403, 1909.
29. Hukuhara, T., and T. Miyake. The intrinsic reflexes in the colon. *Jap. J. Physiol.* **9**: 49–55, 1959.
30. Hukuhara, T., S. Kotani, and G. Sato. Effects of destruction of intramural ganglion cells on colon motility: possible genesis of congenital megacolon. *Jap. J. Physiol.* **11**: 635–640, 1961.
31. Ingersoll, E. H., and L. Jones. The effect upon the colon of electrical stimulation of forebrain areas in the cat. *Am. J. Physiol.* **146**: 187–191, 1946.
32. Kern, F. Jr., T. P. Almy, F. K. Abbot, and M. D. Bogdonoff. The motility of the distal colon in non-specific ulcerative colitis. *Gastroenterology* **19**: 492–503, 1951.
33. Kern, F., Jr., and T. P. Almy. The effects of acetylcholine and methacholine upon the human colon. *J. Clin. Invest.* **31**: 555–560, 1952.
34. Kock, N. G., L. Hulten, and L. Leandoer. A study of the motility in different parts of the human colon. *Scand. J. Gastroent.* **3**: 163–169, 1968.
35. Kohler, R. Evacuation of the normal large intestine. *Acta Radiol.* 2 (diagnosis): 9–16, 1964.
36. Lipkin, M., T. P. Almy, and B. M. Bell. Pressure-volume characteristics of the human colon. *J. Clin. Invest.* **41**: 1831–1839, 1962.
37. Misiewicz, J. J., S. L. Waller, and M. Eisner. Motor responses of human gastrointestinal tract to 5-hydroxytryptamine in vivo and in vitro. *Gut* **7**: 208–216, 1966.
38. Misiewicz, J. J., A. M. Connell, and F. A. Pontes. Comparison of the effects of meals and prostigmine on the proximal and distal colon in patients with and without diarrhoea. *Gut* **7**: 468–473, 1966.
39. Murrell, T. G. C., and A. G. Wangel, and D. J. Deller. Intestinal motility in man. IV. Effect of serotonin on intestinal motility in subjects with diarrhea and constipation. *Gastroenterology* **51**: 656–663, 1966.
40. Murrell, T. G. C., and D. J. Deller. Intestinal motility in man: The effect of bradykinin on the motility of the distal colon. *Am. J. Dig. Dis.* **12**: 568–576, 1967.
41. Nakayama, K., K. Yamamoto, T. Tamiya, H. Makino, M. Odaka, M. Ohwade, and H. Takahashi. Experience with free autographs of the bowel with a new venous anastomosis apparatus. *Surgery* **55**: 796–802, 1964.

42. Neely, J., and B. N. Catchpole. An analysis of the autonomic control of gastro-intestinal motility in the cat. *Gut* **8:** 230–241, 1967.
43. Painter, N. S., S. C. Truelove, G. M. Ardran, and M. Tuckey. Segmentation and the localization of intraluminal pressures in the human colon with special reference to the pathogenesis of colonic diverticula. *Gastroenterology* **49:** 169–177, 1965.
44. Ramorino, M. L., and C. Colagrande. Intestinal motility: Preliminary studies with telemetering capsules and synchronized fluorocinematography. *Am. J. Dig. Dis.* **9:** 64–71, 1964.
45. Reinke, D. A., A. H. Rosenbaum, and D. R. Bennett. Patterns of dog gastro-intestinal contractile activity monitored in vivo with extraluminal force transducers. *Am. J. Dig. Dis.* **12:** 113–141, 1967.
46. Ritchie, J. A., G. M. Ardran, and S. C. Truelove. Motor activity of the sigmoid colon of humans: A combined study by intraluminal pressure recording and cineradiography. *Gastroenterology* **43:** 642–668, 1962.
47. Rosenblum, M. J., and A. J. Cummins. The effect of sleep and of amytal on the motor activity of the human sigmoid colon. *Gastroenterology* **27:** 445–450, 1954.
48. Silva, D. G. Quantitative ultrastructural studies on the nerve fibres in the mucous membrane of the colon. *J. Anat.* **100:** 939–940, 1966.
49. Smith, B. Myenteric plexus in Hirschsprung's disease. *Gut* **8:** 308–312, 1967.
50. Spriggs, E. A., C. F. Code, J. A. Bargen, R. K. Curtiss, and N. C. Hightower, Jr. Motility of the pelvic colon and rectum of normal persons and patients with ulcerative colitis. *Gastroenterology* **19:** 480–491, 1951.
51. Torsoli, A., M. L. Ramorino, and V. Crucioli. The relationships between anatomy and motor activity of the colon. *Am. J. Dig. Dis.* **13:** 462–467, 1968.
52. Truelove, S. C. Movements of the large intestine. *Physiol. Rev.* **46:** 457–512, 1966.
53. Wright, P. G., and J. J. Shepherd. Some observations on the response of normal human sigmoid colon to drugs in vitro. *Gut* **7:** 41–51, 1966.

Motility of the Rectum and Defecation

THE RECTUM exhibits its own characteristic motor activity, but of more importance is the control of the internal and external anal sphincters. Clinical experience indicates that the rectum is usually empty. During defecation, usually a voluntary act, there is an integrated response of the rectum and anal sphincters to accomplish evacuation.

Pressure recordings from the rectum with open-tipped catheters showed very few spontaneous contractions (14) and no basal tone (17). On the other hand, an effective sphincter mechanism at the anus can be demonstrated with a variety of techniques. Open-tipped catheter recordings showed a high-pressure zone reaching a maximum of 45 cm of water 2 to 3 cm above the anal verge (14). The segment was 3 to 5 cm in length. Voluntary contraction of the sphincter increased the pressure 48 cm H_2O above resting levels but this could be sustained for only 50 to 60 seconds (17). This technique for measuring sphincter activity may be misleading. There may be no change over a wide range of pressures in the rectal ampulla (12). By using a catheter with a side aperture, it is possible to measure the pressure necessary to permit a drop of liquid to emerge from the catheter. With such a device, normal resting pressures of 60 to 100 mm of Hg were obtained. These could be increased to 130 to 300 mm with straining to contract the sphincter (13). When the radial force was compared with the pressure within a balloon, increasing intraabdominal pressure by the Valsalva maneuver increased the pressure in the balloon but had little effect on the force gauge. The mucosa may slide over the surface of muscle and change the shape of the balloon (5).

Cineradiographic studies show that the rectum is normally flattened from

199

side to side rather than being cylindrical (*17*). There is a segment above the anus which is usually empty of barium and possibly in a contracted state.

The anal region of man is supplied richly with nerve endings (*7*). While the perianal skin lacks organized nerve endings, the anal canal is supplied abundantly with discrete end knobs, Meissner's corpuscles, Krause end-bulbs, Golgi-Mazzoni bodies, genital corpuscles, and coils and whorls. Above the anal canal the organized nerve endings cease abruptly. Pain, cold, and heat are felt more vividly in the anal canal. There is a correlation between the location of the high-pressure zone and perception of light touch. The anal sphincter extended above the sensory zone in 25 of 27 patients (*6*). Distention of the rectum with a balloon led to relaxation of the sphincter and brought the sensory zone within reach in all subjects. This sensory mechanism probably permits discrimination between flatus and feces in the anal canal.

The sphincter at the anus is composed of an outer, voluntary external sphincter and an inner or internal sphincter composed of smooth muscle. Figure 15-1 illustrates this region together with a recording device for distinguishing contractions from the two components.

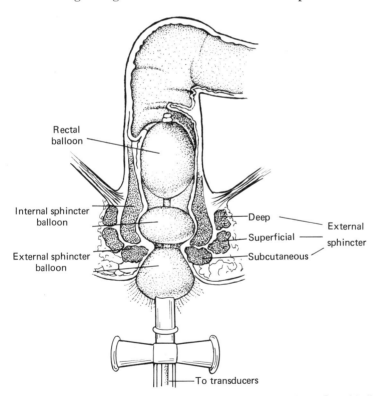

FIGURE 15-1.   Schematic diagram of recording technique. Rectal balloon is shown in distended state used for stimulating changes in sphincter tone. (From M. M. Schuster, F. Hookman, T. R. Hendrix, and A. I. Mendeloff. *Bull. Johns Hopkins Hosp.* **116:** 79–88, © The Johns Hopkins Press, 1965.)

Records of electrical activity in the external anal sphincter indicate that there is tonic activity at rest. Voluntary contraction was associated with vigorous bursts of action potentials, while attempts at defecation were associated with a decrease in activity (9). However, the importance of the external sphincter in maintaining continence may be transient. With patients under succinylcholine, a muscle relaxant, there was little change in sphincter pressures (8).

The nervous control of the external anal sphincter in cats has been well defined (4). Resting electromyographic activity was maintained by either pudendal nerve. Similarly inhibition in response to distention occurred as long as either nerve was intact. Local anesthetics applied to the nerves abolished tonic but not phasic contractions. On the other hand, after clamping the nerve, the phasic responses disappeared first. This suggests that the tonic response is dependent upon smaller nerve fibers. Stimulation of the cut central end of the pudendal nerve was followed by contraction of the sphincter. Afferent traffic in the pudendal nerve decreased with reflex inhibition and increased with phasic responses. Transection of the cord just above the exit of the fourth lumbar nerves abolished both tonic discharge and the inhibitory reflex. Cutting the second sacral dorsal root caused cessation of spontaneous discharge and after cutting S_3, phasic activity stopped. Distention of rectum failed to elicit inhibition of the sphincter after S_2 was cut. Figure 15-2 illustrates the control mechanism.

Stimulation of the presacral nerve in man led to relaxation of the internal sphincter (19). Strips of human internal sphincter contracted when exposed to norepinephrine and relaxed in the pressence of isoprenaline (10). Acetylcholine caused only a small contraction or relaxation in half the experiments.

Distention of the rectum causes relaxation of the anal sphincter unless the distention is applied above the level of a previous transection of the rectum (20). Schuster and his associates (1,15) attempted to differentiate the activity of the internal and external sphincters. They found that distention of the rectum caused relaxation of the internal sphincter but contraction of the external sphincter. They concluded that the internal sphincter may suffice for retaining liquids and flatus. Total internal sphincterotomy reduced sphincteric pressures by 50 per cent. Sensation was also lost, possibly due to scarring (3).

Defecation

Using cineradiography and pressure recordings, the act of defecation can be summarized as follows: The rectum acts as a partially distensible, passive reservoir for feces. Propulsive contractions from the colon cause feces to enter and distend the rectum. During voluntary defecation, there is a rise in intrarectal pressure in response to the general increase in intraabdominal pressure. This forces the walls of the upper portion of the anal canal apart. The descent of the muscles of the pelvic floor pulls the walls of the canal laterally. The

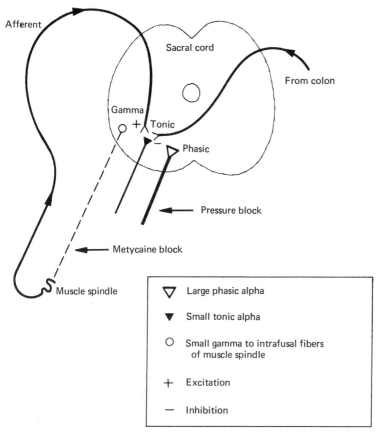

Afferent

Sacral cord

From colon

Gamma

+ Tonic

— Phasic

Pressure block

Metycaine block

Muscle spindle

▽   Large phasic alpha

▼   Small tonic alpha

○   Small gamma to intrafusal fibers
      of muscle spindle

+   Excitation

—   Inhibition

FIGURE 15-2.   Hypothetical scheme for innervation of external anal sphincter. Sphincter receives innervation from three varieties of ventral horn cells. Large alpha phasic cells innervate motor units responsible for vigorous sphincter contractions, phasic responses. Small alpha tonic cells innervate motor units responsible for continuous, resting discharge-tonic response. Very small gamma efferent fibers innervate intrafusal fibers of muscle spindles within sphincter. Sensory endings within spindle have alpha afferent fibers that synapse within cord in some way to keep small alpha tonic ventral horn cells activated. It is proposed that Metycaine and pressure exert their initial effects at sites indicated by arrows. Afferent fibers known to carry inhibitory impulses from colon are also indicated. (From B. Bishop: *J. Neurophysiol.* **22:** 679–692, 1959.)

anal sphincter relaxes and defecation occurs (*17*). Distention of the rectum with a balloon causes bursts of pressure waves from the small intestine. If the colon has been transected or in the presence of truncal vagotomy, this intestinal activity does not occur (*2*).

Division of the spinal cord above the second sacral segment results in the failure of contraction of the external sphincter when the rectum is distended. Following anterolateral cordotomy the rectum must be distended to much greater levels to produce sensation (*16*). With lesions at the level of S_2 to S_5 the anal sphincter and levator ani become paralyzed and the sphincter is patulous (*11*).

The central nervous system at the level of the medulla may also exert a control over defecation. Destruction of areas in the medulla abolishes defecation after the intravenous injection of codeine (*15*).

Pathophysiology

The presence of fecal incontinence correlated closely with low yield pressures at the anal sphincter (*13*). External sphincter activity is normal in Hirschsprung's disease (aganglionosis) (*18*).

References

1. Alva, J., A. I. Mendeloff, and M. M. Schuster. Reflex and electromyographic abnormalities associated with fecal incontinence. *Gastroenterology* **53:** 101–106, 1967.
2. Barany, F. Pressure variations in the rectum and ileum during experimentally induced urgency of defecation. *Acta Med. Scand.* Suppl. **445:** 455–461, 1966.
3. Bennett, R. C., and H. L. Duthie. The functional importance of the internal anal sphincter. *Brit. J. Surg.* **51:** 355–357, 1964.
4. Bishop, B. Reflex activity of external anal sphincter of cat. *J. Neurophysiol.* **22:** 679–692, 1959.
5. Collins, C. D., H. L. Duthie, T. Shelley, and G. E. Whittaker. Force in the anal canal and anal continence. *Gut* **8:** 354–360, 1967.
6. Duthie, H. L., and R. C. Bennett. The relation of sensation in the anal canal to the functional anal sphincter: A possible factor in anal continence. *Gut* **4:** 179–182, 1963.
7. Duthie, H. L., and F. W. Gairns. Sensory nerve-endings and sensation in the anal region of man. *Brit. J. Surg.* **47:** 585–595, 1960.
8. Duthie, H. L., and J. M. Watts. Contribution of the external anal sphincter to the pressure zone in the anal canal. *Gut* **6:** 64–68, 1965.
9. Floyd, W. F., and E. W. Walls. Electromyography of the sphincter ani externus. *J. Physiol.* **122:** 599–609, 1963.
10. Friedmann, C. A. The action of nicotine and catecholamines on the human internal anal sphincter. *Am. J. Dig. Dis.* **13:** 428–431, 1968.
11. Guttmann, L. The regulation of rectal function in spinal paraplegia. *Proc. Roy. Soc. Med.* **52:** 86–89, 1959.
12. Harris, L. D., and C. E. Pope, II. "Squeeze" vs. resistance: An evaluation of the mechanism of sphincter competence. *J. Clin. Invest.* **43:** 2272–2278, 1964.
13. Harris, L. D., C. S. Winans, and C. E. Pope, II. Determination of yield pressures: A method for measuring anal sphincter competence. *Gastroenterology* **50:** 754–760, 1966.

14. Hill, J. R., M. L. Kelley, Jr., J. F. Schlegel, and C. F. Code. Pressure profile of the rectum and anus of healthy persons. *Dis. Colon Rectum* **3:** 203–209, 1960.
15. Koppanyi, T. Studies on defecation with special reference to a medullary defecation center. *J. Lab. Clin. Med.* **16:** 225–238, 1930.
16. Nathan, P. W., and M. C. Smith. Spinal pathways subserving defaecation and sensation from the lower bowel. *J. Neurol. Neurosurg. Psychiat.* **16:** 245–256, 1953.
17. Phillips, S. F., and D. A. W. Edwards. Some aspects of anal continence defaecation. *Gut* **6:** 396–406, 1965.
18. Porter, N. J. Megacolon: A physiological study. *Proc. Roy. Soc. Med.* **54:** 1043–1047, 1961.
19. Shepherd, J. J., and P. G. Wright. The response of the internal anal sphincter in man to stimulation of the presacral nerve. *Am. J. Dig. Dis.* **13:** 421–427, 1968.
20. Schuster, M. M., T. R. Hendrix, and A. I. Mendeloff. The internal anal sphincter response: Manometric studies on its normal physiology, neural pathways and alterations in bowel disorders. *J. Clin. Invest.* **42:** 196–207, 1963.
21. Schuster, M. M., P. Hookman, T. R. Hendrix, and A. I. Mendeloff. Simultaneous manometric recording of internal and external anal sphincteric reflexes. *Bull. Johns Hopkins Hosp.* **116:** 79–88, 1965.

16

A Model of the
Enterohepatic Circulation

IN THE PRECEEDING CHAPTERS we have discussed the control of gastrointestinal function in terms of our present understanding. Although there has been some progress in the application of cellular control systems of protein synthesis and membrane phenomena to cells of the digestive tract, it should be apparent that little use has been made of the techniques of system analysis, as noted in the introduction. In this final chapter, we have sought to find a system within the alimentary canal which might become a suitable candidate for such analytical techniques. Even though the quantitative data necessary for the development of differential equations is not yet available, it seemed worthwhile to indicate by means of a block diagram how systems analysis might be applied. In the case of the control of certain cardiovascular and respiratory systems, such an approach has already led to insights and the design of models subject to experimental testing.

For this purpose we have chosen the enterohepatic circulation of bile salts. It is clear that most of the bile salts in bile enter the portal circulation from the lumen of the intestine and return to the liver, where they are transported again into bile by the hepatic parenchymal cells. The small loss of bile salts in the feces is made up by synthesis of bile salts from cholesterol in the liver. Under normal conditions the body pool of bile salts is maintained at a constant level. Some information is available on the concentration of bile salts in bile, intestinal content, and portal venous blood. Interruption of the enterohepatic circulation leads to a significant increase in the synthesis of bile salts by the liver. Therefore, in this system we have the elements of a regulated function to which systems analysis might be applied when the equations for the transport processes involved become available.

Figure 16-1 shows a block diagram of the processes involved in the enterohepatic circulation of bile salts. The fundamental mechanisms by which bile salts enter the lumen of the biliary canaliculus are (a) transport across the hepatic parenchymal cell and (b) synthesis of bile salts within the cell. Under normal circumstances synthesis contributes only the small amount necessary to balance loss in the feces. The greater proportion is contributed by transport from hepatic sinusoids of bile salts returning in portal blood after absorption from the intestines.

Figure 16-2 is a representation of a simplified scheme, taking into account the absorption processes in the jejunum, ileum, and colon, and the synthesis and transport of bile salts by the hepatocyte or hepatic parenchymal cell.

In the flow diagram, we consider as important variables the rate of change with respect to time of the amount of bile salts leaving the bile ducts (dB_B/dt), entering the jejunum (dB_J/dt) and the colon (dB_C/dt), as well as the loss in feces (dB_L/dt). The absorption of bile salts from the intestinal tract yields the variables (dB_{JV}/dt) for the amount per unit time in jejunal venous blood, (dB_{IV}/dt) for ileal venous blood, and (dB_{CV}/dt) for colonic venous blood. The input to the hepatocytes is described by the rate of change of the amount per unit time in the sinusoids, (dB_S/dt).

The output of bile salts from the hepatocytes is determined by the process

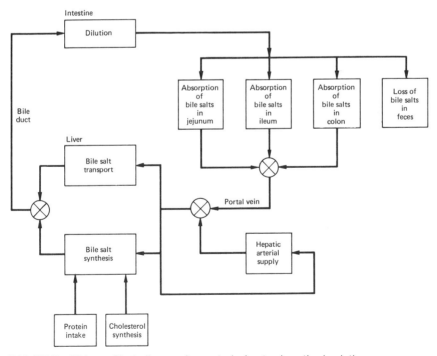

FIGURE 16-1.   Block diagram for control of enterohepatic circulation.

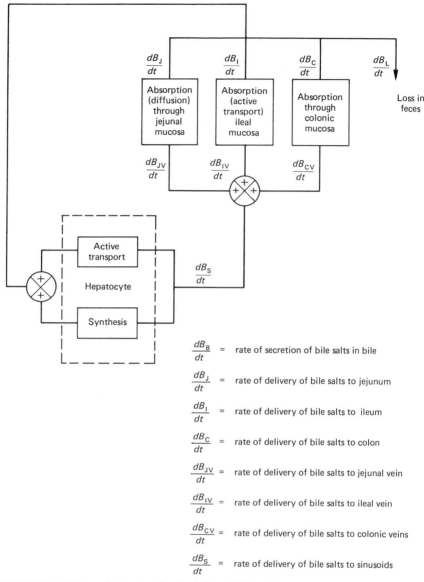

$\dfrac{dB_B}{dt}$ = rate of secretion of bile salts in bile

$\dfrac{dB_J}{dt}$ = rate of delivery of bile salts to jejunum

$\dfrac{dB_I}{dt}$ = rate of delivery of bile salts to ileum

$\dfrac{dB_C}{dt}$ = rate of delivery of bile salts to colon

$\dfrac{dB_{JV}}{dt}$ = rate of delivery of bile salts to jejunal vein

$\dfrac{dB_{IV}}{dt}$ = rate of delivery of bile salts to ileal vein

$\dfrac{dB_{CV}}{dt}$ = rate of delivery of bile salts to colonic veins

$\dfrac{dB_S}{dt}$ = rate of delivery of bile salts to sinusoids

FIGURE 16-2.   Enterohepatic circulation of bile salts.

of synthesis and of transport across the cell membranes and yields the amount of bile salts per unit time in the bile ducts, thus closing the loop.

The synthesis of bile salts is a negative feedback mechanism in the sense that as the rate of delivery of bile salts to the hepatocytes is increased, the rate of synthesis decreases. The transport of bile salts from the sinusoid into the hepatocyte and from hepatocyte to bile is thought to involve active transport processes and is independent of the rate of synthesis, as shown by the results of intravenous taurocholate infusions into bile-salt-depleted animals and those with an intact enterohepatic circulation (2).

The absorption by the jejunal and colonic mucosa is thought to be a passive diffusion phenomenon, whereas absorption by the ileal mucosa is known to involve an active transport mechanism (5).

Figure 16-3 shows Lineweaver-Burk plots for the transport of taurocholate in everted hamster ileal sacs, indicating that Michaelis-Menten relationships hold for the absorption of bile salts in the ileum (4). The apparent k_m value was found to be 1.34 mM and the apparent V_{max} was 10.9 μmoles for a 10-cm sac incubated for 45 minutes. Hence the following relation can be stated:

$$dB_{IV}/dt = 0.12 \times (B_I)/1.34 + (B_I)$$

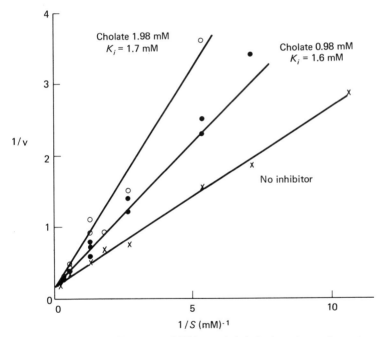

FIGURE 16-3. Transport of S³⁵-taurocholate by hamster seal sacs in presence and absence of sodium cholate (Lineweaver-Burk plots). The taurocholate concentrations in the mucosal media ranged from 0.1 to 7.4 mM. 1/S is the reciprocal of the initial taurocholate concentration. 1/V is the reciprocal of the amount of S³⁵-taurocholate disappearing from the mucosal medium. The lowermost line is for uninhibited taurocholate transport; each point is the mean of 2 to 8 experiments. The upper two lines are for taurocholate transport in the presence of sodium cholate; each point is the result of one experiment. (From M. R. Playoust and K. J. Isselbacher. *J. Clin. Invest.* **43:** 471, 1964.)

where B_I is the concentration in mM/L delivered to the ileum and the rate dB_{IV}/dt is in mg per minute.

The synthesis of bile salts by the hepatocytes has been shown to vary manyfold when the enterohepatic circulation has been interrupted (5). However, synthesis cannot reach the level of bile salt production in animals with an intact enterohepatic circulation.

It is not certain what the signal for stimulation of bile salt synthesis is, although the concentration or rate of delivery of bile salts in sinusoidal blood has been suggested (1). It would be helpful to determine the quantitative effects on bile salt secretion in bile, in animals with an interrupted enterohepatic circulation, of varying the concentration and/or rate of delivery of bile salts in portal blood.

The transport of bile salts from sinusoidal blood to bile accounts for the majority of bile salts in bile in animals with an intact enterohepatic circulation. The 18-mg bile salt pool in the rat has been estimated to circulate ten times a day, while the daily loss of bile salts in rat feces has been estimated as about 30 mg (5). In a steady state an equal amount would be synthesized by the liver to maintain the body pool of bile salts.

There is some evidence that the transport of bile salts from sinusoid to bile canaliculus involves active transport; unfortunately, quantitative information that would permit the determination of velocity constants for the reactions involved is lacking. Such constants would be essential to the development of a mathematical model concerned with the dynamics of the system. Hofmann has commented on the advantages of such an approach (3). We hope that one of the results of this preliminary discussion will be to stimulate investigators to design experiments to provide the quantitative data required.

To test a system model, the response to forcing under experimental conditions can be compared with that of the model due to analogous mathematical forcing. As input or forcing step functions, infusions of important choleretics and the time course of the response followed experimentally and computed have predictive value. The design of such experiments will pinpoint the need for further experiments to obtain more quantitative information about the system.

References

1. Bergstrom, S., and H. Danielsson. Formation and metabolism of bile acids. In: *Handbook of Physiology*, Section 6: Alimentary Canal. Vol. V: Bile; Digestion; Ruminal Physiology. Edited by C. F. Code. Washington, D.C.: American Physiological Society, 1968, pp. 2391–2407.
2. Brooks, F. P., and M. I. Grossman. Unpublished data.
3. Hofmann, A. F. Functions of bile in the alimentary canal. In: *Handbook of Physiology*. Section 6: Alimentary Canal. Vol. V: Bile; Digestion; Ruminal Physiology.

Edited by C. F. Code. Washington, D.C.: American Physiological Society, 1968. pp. 2507–2533.

4. Playoust, M. R., and K. J. Isselbacher. Studies on the transport and metabolism of conjugated bile salts by intestinal mucosa. *J. Clin. Invest.* **43:** 467–476, 1964.

5. Weiner, L. M., and L. Lack. Bile salt absorption; enterohepatic circulation. In: *Handbook of Physiology.* Section 6: Alimentary Canal. Vol. III: Intestinal Absorption. Edited by C. F. Code. Washington, D.C.: American Physiological Society, 1968, pp. 1439–1455.

Index

£3-0-0